ARTIFICIAL INTELLIGENCE AND MEDICINE

VOLUME 2: CLINICAL APPLICATIONS BEFORE THE AVAILABILITY OF CHAT-GTP4

A book in the Modern Medicine series

Kerry Atkinson and Jim Severino

About this book

All the text was written by the authors. Figure 1 is in the public domain. Attribution of Figure 2 is given as per its creator's directions.

Key words: artificial intelligence; machine learning; deep learning; medicine; big data; practical clinical applications

Other books by Kerry Atkinson

Medical books

1. Graft-versus-Host Disease. Editors, S Burakoff, H J Deeg, J Ferrara, K Atkinson. Marcel Dekker Inc, New York, 1990.
2. Clinical Bone Marrow Transplantation. First edition. Editor, K Atkinson. Cambridge University Press, Cambridge UK, 1994.
3. The BMT Data Book: A Manual for Bone Marrow and Blood Stem Cell Transplantation. K. Atkinson, Cambridge University Press, Cambridge UK, 1998.
4. Clinical Bone Marrow and Blood Stem Cell Transplantation. Second Edition. Editor, K. Atkinson. Cambridge University Press, Cambridge UK, 2000.
5. Clinical Bone Marrow and Blood Stem Cell Transplantation. Third Edition. Eds, K. Atkinson, R Champlin, J Ritz, M Brenner, P Ljungman and W Fibbe. Cambridge University Press, Cambridge UK, 2004.
6. The BMT Data Book. Second edition. R Munker, HM Lazarus and K. Atkinson, Cambridge University Press, Cambridge UK, 2009.

7. The BMT Data Book: Including Cellular Therapy. Third edition. R Munker, C Hildebrandt, HM Lazarus and K. Atkinson, Cambridge University Press, Cambridge UK. 2013.

8. Hematopoietic Cell Transplants: Concepts, Controversies and Future Directions. Eds HM Lazarus, RP Gale, A Keating, A Bacigalupo, R Munker, K Atkinson, A Syed. Cambridge University Press, Cambridge, UK. 2017.

9. The Biology and Therapeutic Application of Mesenchymal Cells. Ed. K Atkinson. Wiley/Blackwell. 2017

10. Revolutionizing Tropical Medicine. Eds. K Atkinson and D Mabey. Wiley/Blackwell Publishers Inc. 2019.

11. Asthma: Targeted Biological Treatments 2020. Kindle Direct Publishing, 2020. e-book and paperback

12. Atopic Dermatitis: Targeted Biological Treatments 2020. Kindle Direct Publishing, 2020. e-book and paperback

13. Psoriasis: Targeted Biological Treatments 2020. Kindle Direct Publishing, 2020. e-book and paperback

14. Crohn's disease and ulcerative colitis: Targeted Biological Treatments 2020. Kindle Direct Publishing, 2020. e-book and paperback

15. Rheumatoid arthritis, Juvenile Idiopathic Arthritis, Ankylosing spondylitis, Psoriatic Arthritis and Gout: Targeted Biological Treatments 2020. Kindle Direct Publishing, 2020. e-book and paperback

16. Small Cell Lung Cancer: Targeted Biological Treatments 2020. Kindle Direct Publishing, 2020. e-book and paperback

17. Chronic Myeloid Leukemia: Targeted Biological Treatments 2020. Kindle Direct Publishing, 2020. e-book and paperback

18. Melanoma: Targeted Biological Treatments 2020, Kindle Direct Publishing 2020. e-book and paperback

19. Dementia - A Caregiver's Guide. Kindle Direct Publishing 2020. e-book

20. Breast Cancer: Targeted Biological Treatments 2021. Kindle Direct Publishing 2021. e-book and paperback

21. Non-melanoma Skin Cancers: Targeted Biological and Specifically Designed Therapeutic agents. 2022. Kindle Direct Publishing 2021. e-book and paperback

22. Hodgkin Lymphoma: Targeted Biological Treatments. 2022. Kindle Direct Publishing 2022. e-book and paperback

23. Chimeric Antigen Receptor (CAR) T Cells: The second Revolution in Cellular Therapy. 2022. Kindle Direct Publishing 2022. e-book and paperback

24. Acute lymphoblastic leukemia: targeted immune therapeutic agents. Kindle Direct Publishing 2023. e-book and paperback

25. Artificial Intelligence and Medicine. A book in the Modern Medicine series. Kindle Direct Publishing 2024. e-book and paperback

Natural history/conservation books

26. Bird facts for everyone. K Atkinson. Outskirts Press Inc., Denver, USA. 2014

27. Birds, Birds, Birds. Kindle Direct Publishing 2020. e-book and paperback

28. A Field Guide to the Wild Habitats of Sydney Australia. Kindle Direct Publishing 2021. e-book and paperback

29. Conserving New Zealand's Endangered Species. Kindle Direct Publishing 2021. e-book and paperback

30. Conserving Australia's Endangered Species. Kindle Direct Publishing 2021. e-book and paperback

31. Nature's Wonders: Britain and Ireland. Kindle Direct Publishing 2021. e-book and paperback.

32. Nature's Wonders: Spain and Bulgaria. Kindle Direct Publishing 2022. e-book and paperback.

33. Nature's Wonders: France's Camargue, the Swiss National Park and Portugal. Kindle Direct Publishing 2022. e-book and paperback.

34. Nature's Wonders: Cuba. Kindle Direct Publishing 2022. e-book and paperback.

35. Nature's Wonders: Japan in Winter Kindle Direct Publishing 2022. e-book and paperback.

36. Nature's Wonders: India. Kindle Direct Publishing 2022. e-book and paperback.

37. Nature's Wonders: Tanzania. Kindle Direct Publishing 2022. e-book and paperback.

38. The Silk Road: Uzbekistan and Kazakhstan – A Book in the Nature's Wonders Series. 2022. Kindle Direct Publishing 2022. e-book and paperback.

39. Madagascar – Land of Lemurs and Chameleons: a book in the Nature's Wonders series 2023. Kindle Direct Publishing 2022. e-book and paperback.

40. South Africa - Kalahari to the Cape - a book in the Nature's Wonders series. Kindle Direct Publishing 2022. e-book and paperback

41. Nature's Wonders – Finland - land of owls and lakes. Kindle Direct Publishing 2023. e-book and paperback

42. Nature's Wonders – Ethiopia. Kindle Direct Publishing 2023. e-book and paperback

43. Nature's Wonders – Kakadu National Park and Central Australia. Kindle Direct Publishing 2023. e-book and paperback

44. Nature's Wonders – Lord Howe Island, Australia. Kindle Direct Publishing 2023. e-book and paperback

45. Norway above the Arctic Circle in March. A book in the Nature's Wonders series. Kindle Direct Publishing 2024. e-book and paperback

46. The Inside Passage and the Pribilof Islands. A book in the Nature's Wonders series. Kindle Direct Publishing 2024. e-book and paperback

47. Orca! (and some interesting bird species in Washington State). Kindle Direct Publishing 2024. e-book

Other books

48. Paintings by Kerry Atkinson 2019 – 2021. Kindle Direct Publishing 2021. e-book and paperback.

49. Ferrari Road Cars. Kindle Direct Publishing 2022. e-book and paperback.
50. Paintings by Kerry Atkinson 2022. Kindle Direct Publishing 2022. e-book and paperback.
51. Samuel Beckett and Bob Dylan – living in a Shakespearean era. Kindle Direct Publishing 2022. e-book and paperback.
52. Paintings and sculptures by Kerry Atkinson 2023. Kindle Direct Publishing 2023. e-book and paperback.
53. Ten influential European paintings. Kindle Direct Publishing 2023. e-book and paperback
54. The Pillars of Rock 'N Roll. Kindle Direct Publishing 2024. e-book and paperback
55. Early 20th century western paintings - a smorgasbord of color and radical shapes. Kindle Direct Publishing 2024. e-book and paperback
56. Insects and other wildlife included in Dutch flower paintings from the Dutch golden age. Kindle Direct Publishing 2024. e-book and paperback

TABLE OF CONTENTS

Authors' preface to previous book "Artificial intelligence and Medicine"

Key events in the 20th Century include the two World Wars, the development of nuclear weapons and their use on Hiroshima and Nagasaki, the invention of the jet engine which led to mass global travel, and the invention of the internet and search engines allowing access to information on practically everything, as long as you have a computer or a smartphone, and an internet provider. Learning to use the internet takes about 1 minute and you do not need to know anything about the computer science underlying it.

Another major event spanning the 20th and 21st Centuries is the development and application of artificial intelligence.

Artificial intelligence is the use of large data bases to solve complex problems.

The concept was born in 1956 and The Journal of Artificial Intelligence was first published in 1993. In 2024 The New England Journal of Medicine started to publish a separate sister journal called NEJM AI. The USA Food and Drug Administration (FDA) has approved more than 200 commercial radiology AI products.

Like all technical sciences AI involves a large number of jargon terms. The meaning of many of these is not immediately straightforward to most medical practitioners but are so essential to understanding AI and how it works that we have included a glossary of terms used in machine learning and in AI at the beginning of this book (Chapter 1), rather than at the end of it.

Progress on the use of AI got a major boost in 2022 when ChatGPT-4 (Chat Generative Pre-trained Transformer) was released using freely available software. Chat GPT-4 is a chatbot developed by the software company OpenAI. (A chatbot is a software application or web interface that is designed to mimic human conversation through text or voice interactions). Modern chatbots are typically online and use generative artificial intelligence systems that are capable of maintaining a conversation with a user in natural language and simulating the way a human would behave as a conversational partner. Such chatbots often use deep learning and natural language processing, but simpler chatbots have existed for decades. Based on a large language model, users of ChatGPT-4 can refine and steer a conversation towards a desired length, format, style, level of detail, and language. Successive prompts and replies, known as prompt engineering, are considered at each conversation stage as a context. By January 2023 it had become what was then the fastest-growing consumer software application in history, gaining over 100 million users and contributing to OpenAI's valuation growing to $29 billion. Other major technology companies working in AI include Microsoft, Alphabet

(Google's parent company), Meta (the parent company of Facebook and Instagram) and Amazon.

A word about the brain of mammals, specifically the neocortex, which is the most recent part of the mammalian brain to evolve, is appropriate here, since this is what AI is trying to mimic: the mammalian neocortex is a remarkably complex organ. It is composed by six layers of neurons and appears to be a distinguishing feature of mammals. It covers the whole of the brain and is responsible for connecting each part of the brain with every other part of the brain. It contains many neuronal cell types, oligodendrocytes, and glia, together accounting for over 10 billion cells in the human brain, that form perhaps 10^{13} - 10^{15} intricate connections (synapses) with other regions of the central nervous system. In its human form the neocortex exists at its most complex and evolved state. It is the region of the brain responsible for sensation, action, cognition, and consciousness.

AI is a complex science involving computer science, electrical engineering, mechanical engineering, mathematics, statistics, robotics, biology and linguistics. There are still many things that machines cannot do, such as understanding the nuances of language, common-sense reasoning, and learning a new skill from just one or two examples. AI software will need to master tasks like these if it is to get close to the multifaceted, adaptable, and creative intelligence of humans.

The impact of AI on human activity will be huge, none more so than in medical diagnosis and treatment. AI is now ubiquitous. It is at the core of Google, Alexa, Siri, Cortana, Facebook, Tesla and AlphaGo. A search on Google showed 105 million entries and counting. Google Trends shows a growing demand for this search term consistent with the exponential rise of deep learning.

As well as medicine, cellular biology and molecular biology, doctors will need to understand the use of AI and will likely incorporate it into their practice.

Authors' preface to this book

Our previous book "Artificial Intelligence and Medicine", published by Kindle Direct Publishing, largely explored the *potential* of artificial intelligence (AI) in medicine. That potential is now becoming a reality in clinical practice. This book describes the early results of this reality using AI systems developed before the introduction and availability of CHAT-GPT4, an AI software system built using a large language model.

A large number of jargon terms are used in AI and machine learning (ML), the meaning of which may not be immediately obvious to clinicians. Therefore, the first two chapters from the earlier book have been reproduced in this book. The first chapter of this book defines the terms used in AI and ML. The second chapter of this book is a general introduction to AI and ML. Subsequent chapters in this book describe the practical applications of AI that have already appeared in a number of peer-reviewed papers published in the medical and scientific literature over the last four years. It should be noted that these publications were derived using AI systems in use before the publication in 2023 of ChatGPT-4 and the free access to its software allowed by its manufacturer Open AI. This software has markedly energized the broader use of AI and it is likely that more clinical articles using new AI systems, such as that of ChatGPT-4, will be published in the future.

It had been widely anticipated that the first application of AI in medicine would be in specialities that used images frequently. The most obvious such speciality is radiology in which computers could be trained on hundreds of thousands of images from radiographs, computed tomography (CT) scans, positron emission tomography (PET) scans and magnetic resonance imaging (MRI) scans – to determine, for example, whether a specific abnormality was likely to be malignant or non-malignant. This has turned out to be the case. Additionally, it was likely that the commonest diseases would be those first targeted by AI systems. This has also turned out to be the case with a large number of articles dealing with the commoner diseases: in cancer medicine the four commonest tumors are lung cancer, breast cancer, colo-rectal cancer and prostate cancer.

AI involvement in medicine is a major new development that is currently in its infancy.

Chapter 1. Terms used in machine learning and artificial intelligence

Artificial intelligence

AI, sometimes called machine intelligence, is intelligence demonstrated by machines, in contrast to the natural intelligence displayed by humans and other animals. In computer science AI research is defined as the study of "intelligent agents", meaning any device that perceives its environment and takes actions that maximize its chance of successfully achieving its goals. Colloquially, the term "artificial intelligence" is applied when a machine mimics "cognitive" functions that humans associate with other human minds, such as learning and problem solving. The traditional problems (or goals) of AI research include reasoning, knowledge representation, planning, learning, natural language processing, perception and the ability to move and manipulate objects. General intelligence is among the field's long-term goals. Approaches include statistical methods, computational intelligence, and traditional symbolic AI. Many tools are used in AI, including versions of search and mathematical optimization, artificial neural networks, and methods based on statistics, probability and economics. The AI field draws upon computer science, mathematics, psychology, linguistics, philosophy, to mention only a few.

There is no established unifying theory or paradigm that guides AI research. A few of the most long standing questions that have remained unanswered include this: should artificial intelligence simulate natural intelligence by studying psychology or neurobiology?

Machine learning (ML) is a subfield of artificial intelligence (AI) in which computer programs learn automatically from experience without explicit programming instructions. This learning by machines can be supervised, semi-supervised, or unsupervised. In supervised setup, the machine is fed with datasets of problems with the answers. Machines (ie, computers) learn to pick up the correct answer through trial and error. In unsupervised learning, machines analyze input data with no defined answer. The semi-supervised is a hybrid approach that involves both labelled and unlabelled data.

Artificial neural network

Artificial neural networks are flexible mathematical models that use multiple algorithms to identify complex nonlinear relationships within large datasets (analytics). Information enters the artificial neural network through the input layer, which is then fed through the multiple layers of algorithmic processes. These processes are applied according to the weights learned in the machine learning processes. Finally, the processed data come out of the output layer. Artificial neural networks help the machine for deep learning.

Active learning

The computer can only obtain training labels for a limited set of instances, and it also has to optimize its choice of objects for which to label. When used interactively, these can be presented to the user for labelling.

Affective computing - see social intelligence below.

Agent architectures and cognitive architectures

Researchers have designed systems to build intelligent systems out of interacting intelligent agents in a multi-agent system. A hierarchical control system provides a bridge between sub-symbolic AI at its lowest, reactive levels and traditional symbolic AI at its highest levels, where relaxed time constraints permit planning and world modelling. Some cognitive architectures are custom-built to solve a narrow problem; others, such as SOAR (security orchestration, automation and response), are designed to mimic human cognition and to provide insight into general intelligence. Modern extensions of SOAR are hybrid intelligent systems that include both symbolic and sub-symbolic components. SOAR is a software solution that enables security teams to integrate and coordinate separate tools into streamlined threat response workflows. In large organizations, security operations centers (SOCs) rely on numerous tools to track and respond to cyberthreats.

Algorithm

AI revolves around the use of algorithms. An algorithm is a set of unambiguous instructions that a mechanical computer can execute. In mathematics and computer science, an algorithm is an unambiguous specification of how to solve a class of problems. Algorithms can perform calculations, data processing and automated reasoning tasks. An algorithm can be expressed within a finite amount of space and time and in a well-defined formal language for calculating a function. Starting from an initial state and initial input, the instructions describe a computation that, when executed, proceeds through a finite number of well-defined successive states, eventually producing "output" and terminating at a final ending state; some algorithms, known as randomized algorithms, incorporate random input. A complex algorithm is often built on top of other, simpler, algorithms.

Algorithms can be tree-like or in graphic form:

Tree-like algorithm:

Root node = starting point for processing

Branch node = support other branches or leaves

Leaf node = ending point of tree

Graph-like algorithm: unlike binary tree-like agorithms, a graph-like algorithm has a multitude of connections and can connect in any direction.

Domain

The domains in AI include machine learning, deep learning, natural language processing, computer vision, and data science. AI planning typically involves input to a domain model. Such planners are called domain-independent in order to emphasis the fact that they can solve planning problems from a wide range of domains. Examples of the use of such domains are block stacking, logistics, workflow management, and robot task planning. Hence a single domain-independent planner can be used to solve planning problems in all these various domains.

Domains in ML include supervised learning, unsupervised learning, semi-supervised learning, and reinforcement learning.

An artificial neural network (ANN) learning algorithm, usually called "neural network" (NN), is a learning algorithm that is inspired by biological neural networks. Computations are structured in terms of an interconnected group of artificial neurons, processing information using a connectionist approach to computation. Modern neural networks are non-linear statistical data modelling tools. They are usually used to model complex relationships between inputs and outputs, to find patterns in data, or to capture the statistical structure in an unknown joint probability distribution between observed variables.

Ant colony optimization (ACO)

In computer science and operations research, the ant colony optimization algorithm (ACO) is a probabilistic technique for solving computational problems which can be reduced to finding good paths through graphs. Artificial ants stand for multi-agent methods inspired by the behaviour of real ants. The pheromone-based communication of biological ants is often the predominant paradigm used. Combinations of artificial ants and local search algorithms have become a method of choice for numerous optimization tasks such as vehicle routing and internet routing.

Anti-logic or scruffy AI

Scruffy AI ("scruffies") uses any number of different algorithms and methods to achieve intelligent behavior. Scruffies rely on incremental testing to verify their programs and scruffy programming requires large amounts of hand coding or knowledge engineering. Proponents of scruffies have argued that general intelligence can only be implemented by solving a large number of essentially unrelated problems, and that there is no magic bullet that will allow programs to develop general intelligence autonomously.

Artificial general intelligence (AGI)

Artificial neural networks (ANN) or connectionist systems are computing systems vaguely inspired by the biological neural networks that constitute animal brains. Such systems "learn" to perform tasks by considering examples, generally without being programmed with any task-specific rules. For example, in image recognition, they might learn to identify images that contain cats by analyzing images that have been manually labelled as "cat" or "no cat" and using the results to identify cats in other images. They do this without any prior knowledge about cats, e.g., that they have fur, tails, whiskers and cat-like faces. Instead, they automatically generate identifying characteristics from the learning material that they process. An ANN is based on a collection of connected units or nodes called artificial neurons which loosely model the neurons in a biological brain. Each connection, like the synapses in a biological brain, can transmit a signal from one artificial neuron to another. An artificial neuron that receives a signal can process it and then signal additional artificial neurons connected to it. In common ANN implementations, the signal at a connection between artificial neurons is a real number. The connections between artificial neurons are called 'edges'. Artificial neurons and edges typically have a weight that adjusts as learning proceeds. The weight increases or decreases the strength of the signal at a connection. Artificial neurons may have a threshold such that the signal is only sent if the aggregate signal crosses that threshold. Typically, artificial neurons are aggregated into layers. Different layers may perform different kinds of transformations on their inputs. Signals travel from the first layer (the input layer), to the last layer (the output layer), possibly after traversing the layers multiple times.

Artificial neuron

An artificial neuron is a mathematical function conceived as a model of biological neurons in a neural network. Artificial neurons are the elementary units of artificial neural networks. The artificial neuron receives one or more inputs (representing excitatory postsynaptic potentials and inhibitory postsynaptic potentials at neural dendrites) and sums them to produce an output (or activation, representing a neuron's action potential which is transmitted along its axon).

Association rule learning

Association rule learning is a method for discovering interesting relationships between variables in large databases.

Attention

Attention was developed to address the weaknesses of recurrent neural networks, where words in a sentence are slowly processed one at a time. Recurrent neural networks favor more recent words at the end of a sentence while earlier words fade away in volatile neural activations. Attention gives all words equal access to any part of a sentence in a faster parallel scheme and no longer suffers the wait time of serial processing. Earlier uses attached this mechanism to a serial recurrent neural network's language translation system, but later uses in large language models removed the recurrent neural network and relied heavily on the faster parallel attention scheme.

Automated planning and scheduling

Automated planning and scheduling, sometimes denoted as simply AI planning, is a branch of artificial intelligence that concerns the realization of strategies or action sequences, typically for execution by intelligent agents, autonomous robots and unmanned vehicles. Unlike classical control and classification problems, the solutions are complex and must be discovered and optimized in multidimensional space.

Automated reasoning

Automated reasoning is dedicated to understanding different aspects of reasoning. The study of automated reasoning helps produce computer programs that allow computers to reason completely, or nearly completely, automatically.

Backpropagation

Backpropagation, or backward propagation of errors, is an algorithm that is designed to test for errors working back from output nodes to input nodes. It is an important mathematical tool for improving the accuracy of predictions in data mining and machine learning. Backpropagation computes the gradient of a loss function with respect to the weights of the network for a single input–output example, and does so efficiently, computing the gradient one layer at a time, iterating backward from the last layer to avoid redundant calculations of intermediate terms in the chain rule.

Bayesian inference

This is a method of statistical inference in which Bayes' theorem is used to update the probability for a hypothesis as more evidence or information becomes available. Bayesian inference is an important technique in statistics, and especially in mathematical statistics. Bayesian updating is particularly important in the dynamic analysis of a sequence of data. Bayesian inference has found application in a wide range of activities, including science, engineering, philosophy, medicine, sport, and law. In the philosophy of decision theory, Bayesian inference is closely related to subjective probability, often called "Bayesian probability". An example is "If the current patient has a fever, adjust the probability they have influenza in such-and-such way".

Bayesian network

Bayesian network, belief network or directed acyclic graphical model is a probabilistic graphical model that represents a set of random variables and their conditional independencies via a directed acyclic graph (DAG). For example, a Bayesian network could represent the probabilistic relationships between diseases and symptoms. Given symptoms, the network can be used to compute the probabilities of the presence of various diseases. Efficient algorithms exist that perform inference and learning. A Bayesian network is a type of graphical model that uses probability to determine the occurrence of an event. It is also known as a belief network or a causal network. It consists of directed cyclic graphs (DCGs) and a table of conditional probabilities to find out the probability of an event happening. Bayesian networks are a very general tool that can be used for a large number of problems: reasoning (using the Bayesian inference algorithm), learning (using the expectation-maximization algorithm), planning (using decision networks) and perception (using dynamic Bayesian networks). Probabilistic algorithms can also be used for filtering, prediction, smoothing and finding explanations for streams of data, helping perception systems to analyze processes that occur over time. Compared with symbolic logic, formal Bayesian inference is computationally expensive. For inference to be tractable, most observations must be conditionally independent of one another.

Bayesian probability

This is an interpretation of the concept of probability, in which, instead of frequency or propensity of some phenomenon, probability is interpreted as reasonable expectation representing a state of knowledge or as quantification of a personal belief.

Beam search

This is a heuristic search algorithm that explores a graph by expanding the most promising node in a limited set. Beam search is an optimization of best-first search that reduces its memory requirements. Best-first search is a graph search which orders all partial solutions (states) according to some heuristic. However, in beam search, only a predetermined number of best partial solutions are kept as candidates. Beam search is thus a “greedy” algorithm.

A *heuristic* In mathematical optimization and computer science is a technique designed for problem solving more quickly when classic methods are too slow for finding an exact or approximate solution, or when classic methods fail to find any exact solution in a search space. This is achieved by trading optimality, completeness, accuracy, or precision for speed. In a way, it can be considered a shortcut.

Bees algorithm

This is a population-based search algorithm which mimics the food foraging behaviour of honey bee colonies. In its basic version the algorithm performs a kind of neighbourhood search combined with global search, and can be used for both combinatorial optimization and continuous optimization. The only condition for the application of the bees algorithm is that some measure of topological distance between the solutions is defined. The effectiveness and specific abilities of the bees algorithm have been proven in a number of studies. The biological basis for this is as follows: a colony of honey bees can extend itself over long distances (over 14 km) and in multiple directions simultaneously to harvest nectar or pollen from multiple food sources (flower patches). A small fraction of the colony constantly searches the environment looking for new flower patches. These scout bees move randomly in the area surrounding the hive, evaluating the profitability (net energy yield) of the food sources encountered. When they return to the hive, the scouts deposit the food harvested. Those individuals that found a highly profitable food source go to an area in the hive called the “dance floor”, and perform a ritual known as the waggle dance. Through the waggle dance a scout bee communicates the location of its discovery to idle onlookers, which join in the exploitation of the flower patch. Since the length of the dance is proportional to the scout’s rating of the food source, more foragers get recruited to harvest the best rated flower patches. After dancing, the scout returns to the food source it discovered to collect more food. As long as they are evaluated as profitable, rich food sources will be advertised by the scouts when they return to the hive. Recruited foragers may waggle dance as well, increasing the recruitment for highly rewarding flower patches. Thanks to this autocatalytic process, the bee colony is able to quickly switch the focus of the foraging effort to the most profitable flower patches.

Behavior-based robotics or behavioral robotics

This is an approach in robotics that focuses on robots that are able to exhibit complex-appearing behaviors despite little internal variable state to model its immediate environment, mostly gradually correcting its actions via sensory-motor links. Behavior-based robotics sets itself apart from traditional artificial intelligence by using biological systems as a model. Classic artificial intelligence typically uses a set of steps to solve problems: it follows a path based on internal representations of events compared to the behaviour-based approach. Rather than use preset calculations to tackle a situation, behavior-based robotics relies on adaptability. This advance has allowed behaviour-based robotics to become commonplace in research and data gathering.

Black box

In science, computing, and engineering a black box is a device, system or object which can be viewed in terms of its inputs and outputs (or transfer characteristics), without any knowledge of its internal workings. Its implementation is "opaque" (black). Almost anything might be referred to as a black box: a transistor, an algorithm, or the human brain.

Boids

This is an artificial life program which simulates the flocking behaviour of birds. The name "boid" corresponds to a shortened version of "bird-oid object". As with most artificial life simulations, boids is an example of emergent behavior; that is, the complexity of boids arises from the interaction of individual agents (the boids, in this case) adhering to a set of simple rules. It has been shown that the assumption that each bird in a flock adjusts its velocity and position to the other birds within a fixed radius, the time it takes to converge to a steady state is an iterated exponential of height logarithmic in the number of birds. This means that if the number of birds is large enough, the convergence time will be so great that it might as well be infinite. This result applies only to convergence to a steady state. For example, arrows fired into the air at the edge of a flock will cause the whole flock to react more rapidly than can be explained by interactions with neighbors.

Boolean algebra

This is the branch of algebra in which the values of the variables are the truth values true and false, usually denoted 1 and 0 respectively. Instead of elementary algebra where the values of the variables are numbers, and the prime operations are addition and multiplication, the main operations of Boolean algebra are the conjunction and denoted as ∧, the disjunction or denoted as ∨, and the negation not denoted as ¬. It is thus a formalism for describing logical relations in the same way that ordinary algebra describes numeric relations.

Boolean satisfiability problem

This is sometimes called propositional satisfiability problem and abbreviated as SATISFIABILITY or SAT). It is the problem of determining if there exists an interpretation that satisfies a given Boolean formula. In other words, it asks whether the variables of a given Boolean formula can be consistently replaced by the values TRUE or FALSE in such a way that the formula evaluates to TRUE. If this is the case, the formula is called satisfiable. On the other hand, if no such assignment exists, the function expressed by the formula is FALSE for all possible variable assignments and the formula is unsatisfiable.

Causal calculus

When experimental interventions are not feasible or illegal, the derivation of cause-effect relationship from observational studies must rest on some qualitative theoretical assumptions, for example, that symptoms do not cause diseases, usually expressed in the form of missing arrows in causal graphs such as Bayesian networks

Ceteris paribus or caeteris paribus

This is a Latin phrase meaning "other things equal". English translations of the phrase include "all other things being equal" or "other things held constant" or "all else unchanged". A prediction or a statement about a causal, empirical, or logical relation between two states of affairs is ceteris paribus if it is acknowledged that the prediction, although usually accurate in expected conditions, can fail or the relation can be abolished by intervening factors.

Chlorophyll

This is any of several related green pigments found in cyanobacteria and the chloroplasts of algae and plants. Chloroplasts are organelles (specialized compartments) in plant and algal cells. The main role of chloroplasts is to conduct photosynthesis, in which the photosynthetic pigment chlorophyll captures the energy from sunlight and converts it and stores it in the energy-storage molecules ATP and NADPH while freeing oxygen from water.

Circumscription logic

This is a non-monotonic logic used to formalize the common sense assumption that things are as expected unless otherwise specified.

Classification

Given a population whose members each belong to one of a number of different sets or classes, a classification rule or classifier is a procedure by which the elements of the population set are each predicted to belong to one of the classes. A perfect classification is one for which every element in the population is assigned to the class it really belongs to. Classifiers can be trained in various ways; there are many statistical and machine learning approaches. The decision tree is perhaps the most widely used machine learning algorithm. Other widely used classifiers are the neural network, k-nearest neighbour algorithm, kernel methods such as the support vector machine (SVM), Gaussian mixture model, and the very popular naive Bayes classifier. Classifier performance depends greatly on the characteristics of the data to be classified, such as the dataset size, the dimensionality, and the level of noise. Model-based classifiers perform well if the assumed model is an extremely good fit for the actual data. Otherwise, if no matching model is available, and if accuracy (rather than speed or scalability) is the sole concern, conventional wisdom is that discriminative classifiers (especially SVM) tend to be more accurate than model-based classifiers such as "naive Bayes" on most practical data sets.

Cluster analysis

Cluster analysis is the assignment of a set of observations into subsets (called clusters) so that observations within the same cluster are similar according to some predesignated criterion or criteria, while observations drawn from different clusters are dissimilar. Different clustering techniques make different assumptions on the structure of the data, often defined by some similarity metric and evaluated for example by internal compactness (similarity between members of the same cluster) and separation between different clusters. Other methods are based on estimated density and graph connectivity. Clustering is a method of unsupervised learning, and a common technique for statistical data analysis.

Cognition

This is "the mental action or process of acquiring knowledge and understanding through thought, experience, and the senses". It encompasses processes such as attention, the formation of knowledge, memory, judgment and evaluation, reasoning and "computation", problem solving and decision making, comprehension and production of language. Cognitive processes use existing knowledge and generate new knowledge.

Cognitive simulation AI

The economists Herbert Simon and Allen Newell studied human problem-solving skills and attempted to formalize them; their work laid the foundations of the field of artificial intelligence, as well as cognitive science, operations research and management science. Their research team used the results of psychological experiments to develop programs that simulated the techniques that people used to solve problems. This tradition, centered at Carnegie Mellon University, would eventually culminate in the development of the SOAR architecture in the mid-1980s.

Combinatorial explosion

In mathematics this is the rapid growth of the complexity of a problem due to how the combinatorics of the problem are affected by the input, constraints, and bounds of the problem.

Common sense

This is sound practical judgment concerning everyday matters, or a basic ability to perceive, understand, and judge that is shared by nearly all people. Common sense reasoning is one of the branches of artificial intelligence (AI) that is concerned with simulating the human ability to make presumptions about the type and essence of ordinary situations they encounter every day. These assumptions include judgments about the physical properties, purpose, intentions and behavior of people and objects, as well as possible outcomes of their actions and interactions.

Competitive learning

This is a form of unsupervised learning in artificial neural networks, in which nodes compete for the right to respond to a subset of the input data. A variant of Hebbian learning, competitive learning works by increasing the specialization of each node in the network. It is well suited to finding clusters within data.

Computational computing and soft computing

Computational statistics, or statistical computing is the interface between statistics and computer science. It provides solutions to problems which cannot be solved with complete logical certainty, and where an approximate solution is often sufficient. Other soft computing approaches to AI include fuzzy systems, evolutionary computation and many statistical tools. Computational intelligence and soft computing, including interest in neural networks and "connectionism", was revived by David Rumelhart and others in the middle of the 1980s. Artificial neural networks are an example of soft computing - they are solutions to problems which cannot be solved with complete logical certainty, and where an approximate solution is often sufficient. The application of soft computing to AI is studied collectively by the emerging discipline of computational intelligence.

Computational intelligence

This is the application of soft computing to AI.

Computational learning theory (or just learning theory)

This is a subfield of artificial intelligence devoted to studying the design and analysis of machine learning algorithms.

Computer program

This is a collection of instructions for performing a specific task that is designed to solve a specific class of problems. The instructions of a program are designed to be executed by a computer and it is required that a computer is able to execute programs in order for it to function.

Computer science

This is the study of the theory, experimentation, and engineering that form the basis for the design and use of computers. It is the scientific and practical approach to computation and its applications and the systematic study of the feasibility, structure, expression, and mechanization of the
methodical procedures (or algorithms) that underlie the acquisition, representation, processing, storage, communication of, and access to, information

Computer vision

This is an interdisciplinary field that deals with how computers can be made for gaining high-level understanding from digital images or videos. From the perspective of engineering, it seeks to automate tasks that the human visual system can perform. Computer vision is the ability to analyze visual input. Such input is usually ambiguous; a giant, fifty-meter-tall pedestrian far away may produce exactly the same pixels as a nearby normal-sized pedestrian, requiring AI to judge the relative likelihood and reasonableness of different interpretations, for example by using its "object model" to assess that fifty-meter pedestrians do not exist.

Configuration space

Configuration space is a transformation from the physical space in which the robot is of finite-size into another space in which the robot is treated as a point.

Conjunctive normal form (CNF) is a formula in which a conjunction of one or more clauses occurs, where a clause is a disjunction of literals.

Connectionism is an approach in the fields of cognitive science that hopes to represent mental phenomena using artificial neural networks.

Content delivery network or content distribution network (CDN) is a geographically distributed network of proxy servers and their data centres. The goal is to distribute service spatially relative to end-users to provide high availability and high performance.

Control theory in control systems engineering deals with the control of continuously operating dynamic systems in engineered processes and machines. The objective is to develop a control model for controlling such systems using a control action in an optimum manner without delay or overshoot and ensuring control stability.

Convolutional neural network (CNN, or ConvNet) is a class of deep, feed-forward artificial neural networks, most commonly applied to analyzing visual imagery. CNNs use a variation of multilayer perceptrons designed to require minimal preprocessing. They are also known as shift invariant or space invariant artificial neural networks (SIANN), based on their shared-weights architecture and translation invariance characteristics. Convolutional networks were inspired by biological processes in that the connectivity pattern between neurons resembles the organization of the mammalian visual cortex. Individual cortical neurons respond to stimuli only in a restricted region of the visual field known as the receptive field. The receptive fields of different neurons partially overlap such that they cover the entire visual field. CNNs use relatively little pre-processing compared to other image classification algorithms. This means that the network learns the filters that in traditional algorithms were hand-engineered. This independence from prior knowledge and human effort in feature design is a major advantage. They have applications in image and video recognition, recommender systems and natural language processing. CNNs with 12 convolutional layers were used in conjunction with reinforcement learning by Deepmind's "AlphaGo Lee", the program that beat a top Go champion in 2016.

Central processing unit (CPU)

The CPU is the most important processor in a computer. Its electronic circuitry executes instructions of a computer program, such as arithmetic, logic, controlling, and input/output (I/O) operations. This role contrasts with that of external components, such as main memory and specialized coprocessors such as graphics processing units.

Computer programming languages

Computer programs can be categorized by the programming language paradigm used to produce them. Two of the main paradigms are imperative and declarative.

Imperative languages

Imperative programming languages specify a sequential algorithm using declarations, expressions, and statements:

A *declaration* couples a variable name to a datatype – for example, var x: integer;

An *expression* yields a value – for example, 2 + 2 yields 4

A *statement* might assign an expression to a variable or use the value of a variable to alter the program's control flow – for example: x := 2 + 2; if x = 4 then do something.

One criticism of imperative languages is the side effect of an assignment statement on a class of variables called non-local variables.

Declarative languages

Declarative programming languages describe what computation should be performed and not how to compute it. Declarative programs omit the control flow and are considered sets of instructions. Two broad categories of declarative languages are functional languages and logical languages. The principle behind functional languages (like Haskell) is to not allow side effects, which makes it easier to reason about programs like mathematical functions. The principle behind logical languages (like Prolog) is to define the problem to be solved – the goal – and leave the detailed solution to the Prolog system itself. The goal is defined by providing a list of subgoals. Then each subgoal is defined by further providing a list of its subgoals. If a path of subgoals fails to find a solution, then that subgoal is backtracked and another path is systematically attempted.

Cybernetics is a transdisciplinary approach for exploring regulatory systems—their structures, constraints, and possibilities. Norbert Wiener defined cybernetics in 1948 as "the scientific study of control and communication in the animal and the machine." In the 21st Century, the term is often used in a rather loose way to imply "control of any system using technology." In other words, it is the scientific study of how humans, animals and machines control and communicate with each other.

Cyc and the Japanese Fifth Computer Systems

Cyc is the world's longest-lived artificial intelligence project, attempting to assemble a comprehensive ontology and knowledge base that spans the basic concepts and "rules of thumb" about how the world works (think common sense knowledge but focusing more on things that rarely get written down or said, in contrast with facts one might find somewhere on the internet or retrieve via Google or Wikipedia), with the goal of enabling AI applications to perform human-like reasoning and be less "brittle" when confronted with novel situations that were not preconceived.

Historically, projects such as the Cyc knowledge base (1984 -) and the massive Japanese Fifth Generation Computer Systems initiative (1982 - 1992) attempted to cover the breadth of human cognition. These early projects failed to escape the limitations of non-quantitative symbolic logic models and, in retrospect, greatly underestimated the difficulty of cross-domain AI. Nowadays, the vast majority of current AI researchers work instead on tractable "narrow AI" applications (such as medical diagnosis or automobile navigation).

Cyc knowledge base

Cyc (pronounced syke) is a long-term artificial intelligence project that aims to assemble a comprehensive ontology and knowledge base that spans the basic concepts and rules about how the world works.

Data (plural of datum) are a set of values of qualitative or quantitative variables.

Data analysis, or data analytics, is the process of inspecting, cleansing, transforming, and modelling data with the goal of discovering useful information, informing conclusions, and supporting decision-making.

Data compression is the process of reducing the size of a data file. In signal processing, data compression, source coding, or bit-rate reduction this involves encoding information using fewer bits than the original representation. Compression can be either lossy or lossless. Lossless compression reduces bits by identifying and eliminating statistical redundancy. No information is lost in lossless compression. Lossy compression reduces bits by removing unnecessary or less important information.

Data mining

This is the process of discovering patterns in large data sets involving methods at the intersection of machine learning, statistics, and database systems. Data mining is an interdisciplinary subfield of computer science with an overall goal of extracting information from a data set and transforming the information into a comprehensible structure for further use. Data mining is the analysis step of the "knowledge discovery in databases" process. Aside from the raw analysis step, it also involves database and data management aspects, data preprocessing, model and inference considerations, interestingness metrics, complexity considerations, post-processing of discovered structures, visualization, and online updating. Data mining evolved from the study of pattern recognition and computational learning theory.

Data structure

This refers to a data organization, management and storage format that enables efficient access and modification. More precisely, a data structure is a collection of data values, the relationships among them, and the functions or operations that can be applied to the data.

Davis–Putnam–Logemann–Loveland (DPLL) algorithm is a complete, backtracking-based search algorithm for deciding the satisfiability of propositional logic formulae in conjunctive normal form.

Decision theory (or the theory of choice)

This is the study of the reasoning underlying an agent's choices. Decision theory can be broken into three branches: normative decision theory, which gives advice on how to make the best decisions, given a set of uncertain beliefs and a set of values; descriptive decision theory, which analyzes how existing, possibly irrational agents actually make decisions; and prescriptive decision theory, which tries to guide or give procedures on how or what we should do in order to make best decisions in line with the normative theory.

structures, leaves represent class labels and branches represent conjunctions of features that lead to those class labels.

Decision tree learning

Decision tree learning uses a decision tree as a predictive model, which maps observations about an item to conclusions about the item's target value. Decision tree learning uses a decision tree (as a predictive model) to go from observations about an item (represented in the branches) to conclusions about the item's target value (represented in the leaves). It is one of the predictive modelling approaches used in statistics, data mining and machine learning. Tree models where the target variable can take a discrete set of values are called classification trees; in these tree structures, leaves represent class labels and branches represent conjunctions of features that lead to those class labels

Deep learning algorithms

These discover multiple levels of representation, or a hierarchy of features, with higher-level, more abstract features defined in terms of (or generating) lower-level features. It has been argued that an intelligent machine is one that learns a representation that disentangles the underlying factors of variation that explain the observed data. This approach uses artificial "neurons" that can learn by comparing themselves to the desired output and altering the strengths of the connections between their internal neurons to "reinforce" connections that seemed to be useful. The four main approaches can overlap with each other and with evolutionary systems; for example, neural nets can learn to make inferences, to generalize, and to make analogies. Some systems implicitly or explicitly use multiples of these approaches, alongside many other AI and non-AI algorithms.

Learning algorithms work on the basis that strategies, algorithms, and inferences that worked well in the past are likely to continue working well in the future. These inferences can be obvious, such as "since the sun rose every morning for the last 10,000 days, it will probably rise tomorrow morning as well". Learners also work on the basis of "Occam's razor" (explained above) that the simplest theory that explains the data is the likeliest to be correct. Therefore, to be successful, a learner must be designed such that it prefers simpler theories to complex theories, except in cases where the complex theory is proven substantially better.

Deep learning consists of multiple hidden layers in an artificial neural network. Deep learning is any artificial neural network that can learn a long chain of causal links. For example, a feedforward network with six hidden layers can learn a seven-link causal chain (six hidden layers + output layer) and has a "credit assignment path" (CAP) depth of seven. Many deep learning systems need to be able to learn chains ten or more causal links in length. Deep learning has transformed many important subfields of artificial intelligence, including computer vision, speech recognition, natural language processing and others. The first functional Deep Learning networks were trained one layer at a time. Ivakhnenko's 1971 paper describes the learning of a deep feedforward multilayer perceptron with eight layers, already much deeper than many later networks. In 2006, a publication by Geoffrey Hinton and Ruslan Salakhutdinov introduced another way of pre-training many-layered feedforward neural networks (FNNs) one layer at a time, treating each layer in turn as an unsupervised restricted Boltzmann machine, then using supervised backpropagation for fine-tuning. Similar to shallow artificial neural networks, deep neural networks can model complex non-linear relationships. Over the last few years, advances in both machine learning algorithms and computer hardware have led to more efficient methods for training deep neural networks that contain many layers of non-linear hidden units and a very large output layer. Deep learning often uses convolutional neural networks (CNNs), whose origins can be traced back to the Neocognitron introduced by Kunihiko Fukushima in 1980. In 1989, Yann LeCun and colleagues applied backpropagation to such an architecture. In the early 2000s CNNs processed an estimated 10% to 20% of all the cheques written in the US. Since 2011 fast implementations of CNNs on graphic processing units (GPUs) have won many visual pattern recognition competitions.

Deep recurrent neural networks (RNNs) applied to sequence learning can run arbitrary programs to process arbitrary sequences of inputs. The depth of an RNN is unlimited and depends on the length of its input sequence; thus, an RNN is an example of deep learning. RNNs can be trained by gradient descent but suffer from the vanishing gradient problem. In 1992 it was shown that unsupervised pre-training of a stack of recurrent neural networks can speed up subsequent supervised learning of deep sequential problems. Numerous researchers now use variants of a deep learning recurrent NN called the *long short-term memory* (LSTM) network published by Hochreiter & Schmidhuber in 1997.

Connectionist Temporal Classification (CTC)

At Google, Microsoft and Baidu this approach has revolutionised speech recognition. For example, in 2015 Google's speech recognition experienced a dramatic performance jump of 49% through CTC-trained LSTM, which is now available through Google Voice to billions of smartphone users. Google also used LSTM to improve machine translation. LSTM combined with CNNs also improved automatic image captioning and many other applications.

DeepMind Technologies Limited is a British artificial intelligence company founded in September 2010. The company is based in London, but has research centres in California and Canada. Acquired by Google in 2014, the company has created a neural network that learns how to play video games in a fashion similar to that of humans, as well as a Neural Turing machine, or a neural network that may be able to access an external memory like a conventional Turing machine, resulting in a computer that mimics the short-term memory of the human brain. The company made headlines in 2016 after its AlphaGo program beat a human professional Go player for the first time in October 2015 and again when AlphaGo beat Lee Sedol, the world champion, in a five-game match, which was the subject of a documentary film. A more generic program, AlphaZero, beat the most powerful programs playing go, chess and shogi (Japanese chess) after a few hours of play against itself using reinforcement learning.

Default logic

This is a non-monotonic logic used to formalize reasoning with default assumptions. Default logic can express facts like "by default, something is true"; by contrast, standard logic can only express that something is true or that something is false. This is a problem because reasoning often involves facts that are true in the majority of cases but not in every case.

Density estimation

This is the construction of an estimate, based on observed data, of an unobservable underlying probability density function. The unobservable density function is thought of as the density according to which a large population is distributed; the data are usually thought of as a random sample from that population.

Description logics (DL) are a family of formal knowledge representation languages. Many DLs are more expressive than propositional logic but less expressive than first-order logic. In contrast to the latter, the core reasoning problems for DLs are (usually) decidable, and efficient decision procedures have been designed and implemented for these problems.

Dimensionality reduction, or dimension reduction

This is the process of reducing the number of random variables under consideration by obtaining a set of principal variables. It can be divided into feature selection and feature extraction.

Domain and Application domain

A domain is the targeted subject area of a computer program. Formally it represents the target subject of a specific programming project, whether narrowly or broadly defined. For example, for a particular programming project that has as a goal the creation of a program for a particular hospital, that hospital would be the domain. the project can be expanded in scope to include all hospitals as its domain. In a computer programming design, a domain is defined by delineating a set of common requirements, terminology, and functionality. The word domain is also taken as a synonym of application domain.

Dynamic Bayesian Network (DBN) is a Bayesian network which relates variables to each other over adjacent time steps. This is often called a Two-Timeslice BN (2TBN) because it says that at any point in time T, the value of a variable can be calculated from the internal regressors and the immediate prior value (time T-1).

Economic theory relies upon a priori quantitative economic models, which employ a variety of concepts. The theory typically proceeds with an assumption of *ceteris paribus*, which means holding constant explanatory variables other than the one under consideration. When creating theories, the objective is to find ones which are at least as simple in information requirements, more precise in predictions, and more fruitful in generating additional research than prior theories.

Embodied agents

Also known as interface agents, intelligent agents interact with the environment through a physical body within that environment.

Embodied intelligence

This includes embodied, situated, behaviour-based, and nouvelle AI. Researchers from the related field of robotics rejected symbolic AI and focused on the basic engineering problems that would allow robots to move and survive. This work revived the non-symbolic viewpoint of the early cybernetics researchers of the 1950s and reintroduced the use of control theory in AI. This coincided with the development of the embodied mind thesis in the related field of cognitive science: the idea that aspects of the body (such as movement, perception and visualization) are required for higher intelligence.

Estimation of distribution algorithms (EDAs), sometimes called probabilistic model-building genetic algorithms (PMBGAs), are stochastic optimization methods that guide the search for the optimum by building and sampling explicit probabilistic models of promising candidate solutions. Optimization is viewed as a series of incremental updates of a probabilistic model, starting with the model encoding the uniform distribution over admissible solutions and ending with the model that generates only the global optima.

Eukaryotes are organisms whose cells have a nucleus enclosed within membranes, (unlike prokaryotes such as bacteria and other archaea). Eukaryotic cells also contain other membrane-bound organelles such as mitochondria and the Golgi apparatus, and in addition, some cells of plants and algae contain chloroplasts.

Unlike unicellular archaea and bacteria, eukaryotes may also be multicellular and include organisms consisting of many cell types forming different kinds of tissue.

Event calculus

This is similar to other languages for reasoning about change: the event calculus represents the effects of actions on fluents. However, events can also be external to the system. In event calculus, one can specify the value of fluents at some given time points, the events that take place at given time points, and their effects.

Evolutionary algorithm (EA)

Evolutionary computation is a family of algorithms for global optimization inspired by biological evolution, and the subfield of artificial intelligence and soft computing studying these algorithms. In technical terms, they are a family of population-based trial and error problem solvers with a metaheuristic or stochastic optimization character. Evolutionary computation uses a form of optimization search. For example, they may begin with a population of organisms (the guesses) and then allow them to mutate and recombine, selecting only the fittest to survive each generation (refining the guesses). Classic evolutionary algorithms include genetic algorithms, gene expression programming, and genetic programming. Alternatively, distributed search processes can coordinate via swarm intelligence algorithms. Two popular swarm algorithms used in search are particle swarm optimization (inspired by bird flocking) and ant colony optimization(inspired by ant trails).

Expert systems

These are computer systems that emulate the decision-making ability of a human expert. Expert systems are designed to solve complex problems by reasoning through bodies of knowledge, represented mainly “as if - then rules” rather than through conventional procedural code. The first expert systems were created in the 1970s and then proliferated in the 1980s. Expert systems were among the first truly successful forms of artificial intelligence (AI) software. An expert system is divided into two subsystems: the inference engine and the knowledge base. The knowledge base represents facts and rules. The inference engine applies the rules to the known facts to deduce new facts. Inference engines can also include explanation and debugging abilities.

Explainable AI

Explainability (also referred to as "interpretability") is the concept that a machine learning model and its output can be explained in a way that "makes sense" to a human being at an acceptable level.

Exploratory data analysis (EDA)

This is an approach to analysing data sets to summarize their main characteristics, often with visual methods. A statistical model can be used or not, but primarily EDA is for seeing what the data can reveal beyond the formal modelling or hypothesis testing task.

Extended mind thesis (EMT) states that an agent's mind and associated cognitive processing are neither skull-bound nor even body-bound but extend into the agent's world. Within developmental robotics, developmental learning approaches are elaborated upon to allow robots to accumulate repertoires of novel skills through autonomous self-exploration, social interaction with human teachers, and the use of guidance mechanisms (such as active learning, maturation, and motor synergies).

Falling hardware prices and the development of graphics processing units (GPUs) for personal use in the last few years have contributed to the development of the concept of deep learning. This approach tries to model the way the human brain processes light and sound into vision and hearing. Some successful applications of deep learning are computer vision and speech recognition.

Feature selection approach

Feature selection is the process of selecting an optimal subset of relevant features for use in model construction. It is assumed the data contain some features that are either redundant or irrelevant and can thus be removed to reduce calculation cost without incurring much loss of information. Common optimality criteria include accuracy, similarity and information measures.

Feedforward neural network

This is an artificial neural network wherein connections between the nodes do not form a cycle. As such, it is different from recurrent neural networks. Feedforward neural networks were the first and simplest type of artificial neural network devised. In this network, the information moves in only one direction, forward, from the input nodes, through the hidden nodes (if any) and to the output nodes. There are no cycles or loops in the network. As such, it is different from recurrent neural networks.

Fifth Generation Computer Systems

This was an initiative by Japan's Ministry of International Trade and Industry, begun in 1982, to create a computer using massively parallel computing/processing. It aimed to create an "epoch-making computer" with supercomputer-like performance and to provide a platform for future developments in artificial intelligence.

In the history of computing hardware, computers using vacuum tubes were called the first generation; transistors and diodes, the second; integrated circuits, the third; and those using microprocessors, the fourth. Whereas previous computer generations had focused on increasing the number of logic elements in a single CPU, it was widely believed at the time, that the fifth generation would instead turn to massive numbers of CPUs for added performance.

First-order logic, also known as first-order predicate calculus and predicate logic, is a collection of formal systems used in mathematics, philosophy, linguistics, and computer science. First-order logic uses quantified variables over non-logical objects and allows the use of sentences that contain variables, so that rather than propositions such as "Socrates is a man' one can have expressions in the form "there exists X such that X is Socrates and X is a man". This distinguishes it from propositional logic, which does not use quantifiers or relations. First-order logic adds quantifiers and predicates, and can express facts about objects, their properties, and their relations with each other.

Fitness function is a particular type of objective function that is used to summarise how close a given design solution is to achieving the set aims. Fitness functions are used in genetic programming and genetic algorithms to guide simulations towards optimal design solutions.

Fluent calculus is a formalism for expressing dynamical domains in first-order logic. It is a variant of situation calculus; the main difference is that situations are considered representations of states.

Fluents in artificial intelligence are conditions that can change over time. In logical approaches to reasoning about actions, fluents can be represented in first-order logic by predicates having an argument that depends on time.

Formal language

Formalism is a theory that holds that statements of mathematics and logic can be considered to be statements about the consequences of certain string manipulation rules.

Frame problem in artificial intelligence describes an issue with using *first-order logic* (FOL) to express facts about a robot in the world. Representing the state of a robot with traditional FOL requires the use of many axioms that simply imply that things in the environment do not change arbitrarily. Fuzzy logic is a form of many-valued logic in which the truth values of variables may be any real number between 0 and 1. It is employed to handle the concept of partial truth, where the truth value may range between completely true and completely false. By contrast, in Boolean logic, the truth values of variables may only be the integer values 0 or 1.

Fuzzy logic is successfully used in control systems to allow experts to contribute vague rules such as "if you are close to the destination station and moving fast, increase the train's brake pressure"; these vague rules can then be numerically refined within the system. Fuzzy logic is a fuzzy control system based on fuzzy logic - a mathematical system that analyzes analog input values in terms of logical variables that take on continuous values between 0 and 1, in contrast to classical or digital logic, which operates on discrete values of either 1 or 0 (true or false, respectively).

Fuzzy logic fails to scale well in knowledge bases; many AI researchers question the validity of chaining fuzzy-logic inferences.

Fuzzy set theory assigns a "degree of truth" (between 0 and 1) to vague statements such as "Alice is old" (or rich, or tall, or hungry) that are too linguistically imprecise to be completely true or false. In classical set theory, the membership of elements in a set is assessed in binary terms according to a bivalent condition - an element either belongs or does not belong to the set. By contrast, fuzzy set theory permits the gradual assessment of the membership of elements in a set; this is described with the aid of a membership function valued in the real unit interval – 0 or 1.

Game theory is the study of mathematical models of strategic interaction between rational decision-makers. It has applications in all fields of social science, as well as in logic and computer science. Originally, it addressed zero-sum games, in which one person's gains result in losses for the other participants. Today, game theory applies to a wide range of behavioural relations, and is now an umbrella term for the science of logical decision making in humans, animals, and computers.

Gene expression programming (GEP) is an evolutionary algorithm that creates computer programs or models. These computer programs are complex tree structures that learn and adapt by changing their sizes, shapes, and composition, much like a living organism. And like living organisms, the computer programs of GEP are also encoded in simple linear chromosomes of fixed length. Thus, GEP is a genotype–phenotype system, benefiting from a simple genome to keep and transmit the genetic information and a complex phenotype to explore the environment and adapt to it.

Generalized coordinates: in classical mechanics the parameters that define the configuration of a system are called generalized coordinates, and the vector space defined by these coordinates is called the configuration space of the physical system.

Genetic algorithm (GA) is a search heuristic that mimics the process of natural selection, and uses methods such as mutation and crossover to generate new genotypes in the hope of finding good solutions to a given problem. Conversely, machine learning techniques have been used to improve the performance of genetic and evolutionary algorithms.

Genetic programming (GP) is a technique whereby computer programs are encoded as a set of genes that are then modified (evolved) using an evolutionary algorithm (often a genetic algorithm, (GA); it is an application of genetic algorithms where the space of solutions consists of computer programs. The results are computer programs that are able to perform well in a predefined task. The methods used to encode a computer program in an artificial chromosome and to evaluate its fitness with respect to the predefined task are central in the GP technique.

Genetic recombination (also known as *genetic reshuffling*) is the production of offspring with combinations of traits that differ from those found in either parent. In eukaryotes, genetic recombination during meiosis can lead to a novel set of genetic information that can be passed on from the parents to the offspring. Most recombination is naturally occurring.

Group method of data handling (GMDH) is used in such fields as data mining, knowledge discovery, prediction, complex systems modelling, optimization and pattern recognition.

Golgi apparatus is an organelle found in most eukaryotic cells. Part of the endomembrane system in the cytoplasm, the Golgi apparatus packages proteins into membrane-bound-vesicles inside the cell before the vesicles are sent to their destination. The Golgi apparatus resides at the intersection of the secretory, lysosomal, and endocytic pathways. It is of particular importance in processing proteins for secretion, containing a set of glycosylation enzymes that attach various sugar monomers to proteins as the proteins move through the apparatus.

Gradient descent and *gradient ascent*

This is a first order iterative optimization algorithm for finding the minimum of a function. To find a local minimum of a function using gradient descent, one takes steps proportional to the negative of the gradient (or approximate gradient) of the function at the current point. If instead one takes steps proportional to the positive of the gradient, one approaches a local maximum of that function; the procedure is then known as gradient ascent.

Greedy algorithm is an algorithmic paradigm that follows the problem-solving heuristic of making the locally optimal choice at each stage with the intent of finding a global optimum. In many problems, a greedy strategy does not usually produce an optimal solution, but nonetheless a greedy heuristic may yield locally optimal solutions that approximate a globally optimal solution in a reasonable amount of time.

Hebbian theory is a neuroscientific theory claiming that an increase in synaptic efficacy arises from a presynaptic cell's repeated and persistent stimulation of a postsynaptic cell. It is an attempt to explain synaptic plasticity such as the adaptation of brain neurons during the learning process.

Hidden Markov Model (HMM) is a statistical Markov model in which the system being modelled is assumed to be a Markov process with unobserved (i.e. hidden) states. The hidden Markov model can be represented as the simplest dynamic Bayesian network.

Hierarchical temporal memory (HTM) is a biologically constrained theory (or model) of intelligence. HTM is rigorously based on neuroscience and the physiology and interaction of pyramidal neurons in the neocortex of the mammalian (in particular, human) brain. At the core of HTM are learning algorithms that can store, learn, infer and recall high-order sequences. Unlike most other machine learning methods, HTM learns (in an unsupervised fashion) time-based patterns in unlabelled data on a continuous basis. HTM is robust to noise, and it has high capacity, meaning that it can learn multiple patterns simultaneously. When applied to computers, HTM is well suited for prediction, anomaly detection, classification and ultimately sensorimotor applications. Hierarchical temporal memory is an approach that models some of the structural and algorithmic properties of the neocortex.

Hill climbing is a mathematical optimization technique which belongs to the family of local search. It is an iterative algorithm that starts with an arbitrary solution to a problem, then attempts to find a better solution by making an incremental change to the solution. If the change produces a better solution, another incremental change is made to the new solution, and so on until no further improvements can be found.

Artificial general intelligence

Currently the vast majority of current AI researchers work on tractable "narrow AI" applications (such as medical diagnosis or automobile navigation). Many researchers predict that such "narrow AI" work in different individual domains will eventually be incorporated into a machine with *artificial general intelligence* (AGI), combining narrow skills and at some point even exceeding human ability in most or all these areas. Many advances have general, cross-domain significance. One high-profile example is that DeepMind in the 2010s developed a "generalized artificial intelligence" that could learn many diverse Atari games on its own, and later developed a variant of the system which succeeded at sequential learning.

Besides transfer learning, hypothetical AGI breakthroughs could include the development of reflective architectures that can engage in decision-theoretic meta-reasoning, and figuring out how to "slurp up" a comprehensive knowledge base from the entire unstructured Web. Some argue that some kind of (currently undiscovered) conceptually straightforward, but mathematically difficult, "Master Algorithm" could lead to AGI.

A few "emergent" approaches look to simulating human intelligence extremely closely, and believe that anthropomorphic features like an artificial brain or simulated child development may someday reach a critical point where general intelligence emerges. Many of the problems with this is that it may also require general intelligence, if machines are to solve the problems as well as people do. For example, even specific straightforward tasks, like machine translation, require that a machine read and write in both languages, follow the author's argument (reason), know what is being talked about (knowledge), and faithfully reproduce the author's original intent (social intelligence). A problem like machine translation is considered "AI-complete", because all of these problems need to be solved simultaneously in order to reach human-level machine performance.

In AGI research some researchers caution against over-reliance on statistical learning, and argue that continuing research into GOFAI will still be necessary to attain general intelligence.

Explainable AI (XAI) or *Transparent AI* is an artificial intelligence whose actions can be easily understood by humans. It contrasts with the concept of the "black box" in machine learning, where even their designers cannot explain how the AI arrived at a specific decision. XAI can be used to implement a social right to explanation. Transparency rarely comes for free; there are often trade-offs between how "smart" an AI is and how transparent it is, and these trade-offs are expected to grow larger as AI systems increase in internal complexity. The technical challenge of explaining AI decisions is sometimes known as the interpretability problem.

Labelling

In machine learning, data labelling is the process of identifying raw data (images, text files, videos, etc.) and adding one or more meaningful and informative labels to provide context so that a machine learning model can learn from it.

Noise

In machine learning, noise refers to unwanted behaviours within the data that provide a low signal-to-noise ratio. Noise refers to random or unpredictable fluctuations in data that disrupt the ability to identify target patterns or relationships. The result is decreased accuracy or reliability of a model's predictions or output. Essentially, data = signal + noise. While a minority of the noise in data is irreducible, most can be prevented by understanding its causes and correcting them.

Formal language

This is a set of strings of symbols together with a set of rules that are specific to it.

Inductive logic programming

Inductive logic programming (ILP) is an approach to rule learning using logic programming as a uniform representation for input examples, background knowledge, and hypotheses. Given an encoding of the known background knowledge and a set of examples represented as a logical database of facts, an ILP system will derive a hypothesized logic program that entails all positive and no negative examples. Inductive programming is a related field that considers any kind of programming languages for representing hypotheses such as functional programs.

Inference engines

These are a component of the system that applies logical rules to the knowledge base to deduce new information. The first inference engines were components of expert systems. The typical expert system consisted of a knowledge base and an inference engine. The knowledge base stores facts about the world. The inference engine applies logical rules to the knowledge base and deduced new knowledge. This process would iterate as each new fact in the knowledge base could trigger additional rules in the inference engine. Inference engines work primarily in one of two modes: forward chaining and backward chaining.

Forward chaining and *backward chaining*

This starts with the known facts and asserts new facts. Backward chaining starts with goals and works backward to determine what facts must be asserted so that the goals can be achieved.

Information theory

This studies the quantification, storage, and communication of information. It was originally proposed by Claude E. Shannon in 1948 to find fundamental limits on signal processing and communication operations such as data compression in a landmark paper entitled "A Mathematical Theory of Communication". Applications of fundamental topics of information theory include lossless data compression (e.g. ZIP files), lossy data compression (e.g. MP3s and JPEGs), and channel coding (e.g. for digital subscriber line (DSL)). Information theory studies the quantification, storage, and communication of information.

Integer

An integer is a whole number (not a fractional number) that can be positive, negative, or zero.

Intelligent agent

An intelligent agent is an autonomous entity which observes through sensors and acts upon an environment using actuators (i.e. it is an agent) and directs its activity towards achieving goals (i.e. it is "rational", as defined in economics). Intelligent agents may also learn or use knowledge to achieve their goals. They may be very simple or very complex. A reflex machine, such as a thermostat, is considered an example of an intelligent agent. The simplest intelligent agents are programs that solve specific problems. More complicated agents include human beings and organizations of human beings (such as firms). The paradigm allows researchers to directly compare or even combine different approaches to isolated problems, by asking which agent is best at maximizing a given "goal function". An agent that solves a specific problem can use any approach that works – some agents are symbolic and logical, some are sub-symbolic artificial neural networks and others may use new approaches. The paradigm also gives researchers a common language to communicate with other fields - such as decision theory and economics - that also use concepts of abstract agents. Building a complete agent requires researchers to address realistic problems of integration; for example, because sensory systems give uncertain information about the environment, planning systems must be able to function in the presence of uncertainty. The intelligent agent paradigm became widely accepted during the 1990s. Intelligent agent must be able to set goals and achieve them. They need a way to visualize the future - a representation of the state of the world and be able to make predictions about how their actions will change it - and be able to make choices that maximize the utility (or "value") of available choices. In classical planning problems, the agent can assume that it is the only system acting in the world, allowing the agent to be certain of the consequences of its actions. However, if the agent is not the only actor, then the agent must be able to reason under uncertainty. This calls for an agent that can not only assess its environment and make predictions, but also evaluate its predictions and adapt based on its assessment. Multi-agent planning uses the cooperation and competition of many agents to achieve a given goal. Emergent behavior such as this is used by evolutionary algorithms and swarm intelligence.

k-NN classification

An object is classified by a majority vote of its neighbours, with the object being assigned to the class most common among its k-nearest neighbours (k is a positive integer, typically small). If k = 1, then the object is simply assigned to the class of that single nearest neighbour. In k-NN regression, the output is the property value for the object. This value is the average of the values of its k-nearest neighbours. k-nearest neighbours algorithm is a non-parametric method used in pattern recognition for classification and regression. In both cases the input consists of the k closest training examples in the feature space. The output depends on whether k-NN is used for classification or regression: k-NN is a type of instance-based learning, or lazy learning, where the function is only approximated locally and all computation is deferred until classification. The k-NN algorithm is among the simplest of all machine learning algorithms.

Knowledge bases

These represent a technology used to store complex structured and unstructured information used by a computer system. The initial use of the term was in connection with expert systems which were the first knowledge-based systems.

Knowledge representation and reasoning (KR, KR^2, KR&R)

This is a field of artificial intelligence dedicated to representing information about the world in a form that a computer system can utilize to solve complex tasks such as diagnosing a medical condition or having a dialogue in a natural language. Knowledge representation incorporates findings from psychology about how humans solve problems and represent knowledge in order to design formalisms that will make complex systems easier to design and build. Knowledge representation and reasoning also incorporates findings from logic to automate various kinds of reasoning, such as the application of rules or the relations of sets and subsets. Examples of knowledge representation formalisms include semantic nets, systems architecture, frames, rules, and ontologies. Examples of automated reasoning engines include inference engines, theorem provers, and classifiers. Knowledge representation and knowledge engineering are central to classical AI research. Some expert systems attempt to gather together explicit knowledge possessed by experts in a narrow domain. In addition, some projects have attempted to gather the "commonsense knowledge" known to the average person into a database containing extensive knowledge about the world. Among the things a comprehensive commonsense knowledge base would contain are objects, properties, categories and relations between objects; situations, events, states and time; causes and effects; knowledge about knowledge (what we know about what other people know); and many other, less well researched domains. A representation of "what exists" is an *ontology*: the set of objects, relations, concepts, and properties formally described so that software agents can interpret them. The semantics of these are captured as description logic concepts, roles, and individuals, and typically implemented as classes, properties, and individuals in the Web Ontology Language. The most general ontologies are called upper ontologies, which attempt to provlde a foundation for all other knowledge by acting as mediators between domain ontologies that cover specific knowledge about a particular knowledge domain (field of interest or area of concern). Such formal knowledge representations can be used in content-based indexing and retrieval, scene interpretation, clinical decision support, knowledge discovery (mining "interesting" and actionable inferences from large databases), and other areas.

Knowledge

Much of what people know is not represented as "facts" or "statements" that they could express verbally. For example, a chess master will avoid a particular chess position because it "feels too exposed" or an art critic can take one look at a statue and realize that it is a fake. These are non-conscious and sub-symbolic intuitions or tendencies in the human brain. Knowledge like this informs, supports and provides a context for symbolic, conscious knowledge. As with the related problem of sub-symbolic reasoning, it is hoped that situated AI, computational intelligence, or statistical AI will provide ways to represent this kind of knowledge.

Knowledge-based AI

When computers with large memories became available around 1970, researchers began to build knowledge into AI applications. This "knowledge revolution" led to the development and deployment of expert systems, the first truly successful form of AI software. The knowledge revolution was also driven by the realization that enormous amounts of knowledge would be required by many simple AI applications.

Large language model (LLM)

Large language model is a type of language model notable for its ability to achieve general-purpose language understanding and generation. LLMs acquire these abilities by using massive amounts of data to learn billions of parameters during training and consuming large computational resources during their training and operation. LLMs are artificial neural networks (mainly transformers) and are (pre-) trained using self-supervised learning and semi-supervised learning.

Learning classifier systems

Learning classifier systems (LCS) are a family of rule-based machine learning algorithms that combine a discovery component (e.g. typically a genetic algorithm) with a learning component (performing either supervised learning, reinforcement learning, or unsupervised learning). They seek to identify a set of context-dependent rules that collectively store and apply knowledge in a piecewise manner in order to make predictions.

Learning to learn, or meta learning

This is a subfield of machine learning in which automatic learning algorithms are applied to metadata about machine learning experiments. The main goal is to use such metadata to understand how automatic learning can become flexible in solving learning problems in order to improve the performance of existing learning algorithms or to learn (induce) the learning algorithm itself.

Metadata

Metadata is "data that provides information about other data", but not the content of the data itself, such as the text of a message or the image itself. There are many distinct types of metadata.

Learning to rank or machine-learned ranking (MLR)

This is the application of machine learning, typically supervised, semi-supervised or reinforcement learning, in the construction of ranking models for information retrieval systems

Lidar (also called LIDAR, LiDAR, and LADAR)

This is a surveying method that measures distance to a target by illuminating the target with pulsed laser light and measuring the reflected pulses with a sensor. Differences in laser return times and wavelengths can then be used to make digital 3-D representations of the target. The name lidar, now used as an acronym of light detection and ranging (sometimes light imaging, detection, and ranging), was originally a portmanteau of light and radar. Lidar is sometimes called laser scanning and 3-D scanning, with terrestrial, airborne and mobile applications.

Logic

This is used for knowledge representation and problem solving, but it can be applied to other problems as well. For example, the satplan algorithm uses logic for planning and inductive logic programming is a method for learning. (Satplan (also known as Planning as Satisfiability) is a method for automated planning. It converts the planning problem instance into an instance of the Boolean satisfiability problem, which is then solved using a method for establishing satisfiability such as the DPLL algorithm or WalkSAT). Logic consists of the systematic study of the form of valid inference. A valid inference is one where there is a specific relation of logical support between the assumptions of the inference and its conclusion. In ordinary discourse, inferences may be signified by words like therefore, hence, and ergo. Logic originally meant "the word" or "what is spoken", but is coming to mean "thought" or "reason" and is a subject concerned with the most general laws of truth, and is now generally held to consist of the systematic study of the form of valid inference. A valid inference is one where there is a specific relation of logical support between the assumptions of the inference and its conclusion.

Logic-based AI

John McCarthy felt that machines did not need to simulate human thought, but should instead try to find the essence of abstract reasoning and problem-solving, regardless of whether people used the same algorithms. His laboratory at Stanford University focused on using formal logic to solve a wide variety of problems, including knowledge representation, planning and learning. Logic was also the focus of work at the University of Edinburgh and elsewhere in Europe which led to the development of the programming language Prolog and the science of logic programming.

Long short-term memory (LSTM)

These are units of a recurrent neural network (RNN). An RNN composed of LSTM units is often called an LSTM network. A common LSTM unit is composed of a cell, an input gate, an output gate and a forget gate. The cell remembers values over arbitrary time intervals and the three gates regulate the flow of information into and out of the cell. LSTM networks are well-suited to classifying, processing and making predictions based on time series data, since there can be lags of unknown duration between important events in a time series. LSTMs were developed to deal with the exploding and vanishing gradient problems that can be encountered when training traditional RNNs

Loss of function.

Loss function or cost function in mathematical optimization, statistics, econometrics, decision theory, machine learning and computational neuroscience, is a function that maps an event or values of one or more variables onto a real number intuitively representing some "cost" associated with the event. An optimization problem seeks to minimize a loss function. An objective function is either a loss function or its negative (in specific domains, variously called a reward function, a profit function, a utility function or a fitness function), in which case it is to be maximized.

Lossless compression

This is a class of data compression algorithms that allows the original data to be perfectly reconstructed from the compressed data.

Lossy compression

This permits reconstruction only of an approximation of the original data, though usually with improved compression rates (and therefore reduced file sizes).

Machine learning

A categorization of machine learning tasks arises when one considers the desired output of a machine-learned system. Machine learning tasks are typically classified into two broad categories, depending on whether there is a learning "signal" or "feedback" available to a learning system. Machine learning is a subset of artificial intelligence in the field of computer science that often uses statistical techniques to give computers the ability to "learn" (i.e., progressively improve performance on a specific task) with data, without being explicitly programmed. Machine learning-based attention is a mechanism mimicking cognitive attention. It calculates "soft" weights for each word, more precisely for its embedding, in the context window. It can do it either in parallel (such as in transformers) or sequentially (such as recurrent neural networks). "Soft" weights can change during each runtime, in contrast to "hard" weights, which are (pre-)trained and fine-tuned and remain frozen afterwards.

Machine perception

This is the ability to use input from sensors (such as cameras (visible spectrum or infrared), microphones, wireless signals, and active lidar, sonar, radar, and tactile sensors) to deduce aspects of the world. Applications include speech recognition, facial recognition, and object recognition. Machine perception is the capability of a computer system to interpret data in a manner that is similar to the way humans use their senses to relate to the world around them. The basic method that the computers take in, and respond to, their environment is through the attached hardware. Until recently input was limited to a keyboard, or a mouse, but advances in technology, both in hardware and software, have allowed computers to take in sensory input in a way similar to humans.

Many of the things people know take the form of "working assumptions". For example, if a bird comes up in conversation, people typically picture a creature that is fist-sized, sings, and flies. None of these things are true about all birds. This problem was identified in 1969 as the qualification problem: for any commonsense rule that AI researchers care to represent, there tend to be a huge number of exceptions. Almost nothing is simply true or false in the way that abstract logic requires. AI research has explored a number of solutions to this problem. Many problems in AI (in reasoning, planning, learning, perception, and robotics) require the agent to operate with incomplete or uncertain information. AI researchers have devised a number of powerful tools to solve these problems using methods from probability theory and economics.

Manifold learning algorithms (Markov process)

Markov process, named after the Russian mathematician Andrey Markov, is a stochastic process that satisfies the Markov property (sometimes characterized as "memorylessness"). Roughly speaking, a process satisfies the Markov property if it can make predictions for the future of the process based solely on its present state just as well as it could knowing by knowing the process's full history.

Massively parallel

This is a term which refers to the use of a large number of processors (or separate computers) to perform a set of coordinated computations in parallel (simultaneously).

Mathematical optimization or mathematical programming

This is the selection of a best element (with regard to a specific criterion) from some set of available alternatives.

Means-ends analysis (MEA) is a problem-solving technique used commonly in artificial intelligence for limiting search in AI programs.

Meiosis

Meiosis is a specialized type of cell division that reduces the chromosome number by half, creating four haploid cells, each genetically distinct from the parent cell that gave rise to them. This process occurs in all sexually reproducing single-celled and multicellular eukaryotes, including animals, plants, and fungi. Meiosis is a special type of cell division of germ cells in sexually-reproducing organisms that produces the gametes - sperm or egg cells.

Metaheuristic

This is a higher-level procedure or a heuristic designed to find, generate, or select a heuristic (partial search algorithm) that may provide a sufficiently good solution to an optimization problem, especially with incomplete or imperfect information or limited computation capacity. Metaheuristics sample a set of solutions which is too large to be completely sampled. Metaheuristics may make few assumptions about the optimization problem being solved, and so they may be usable for a variety of problems.

Methodological individualism

This is the requirement that causal accounts of social phenomena explain how they result from the motivations and actions of individual agents, at least in principle.

Mitochondria

These are double-membrane-bound organelles found in most eukaryotic organisms. Mitochondria generate most of the cell's supply of adenosine triphosphate (ATP), used as a source of chemical energy. Mitochondria are commonly between 0.75 and 3 μm in diameter but vary considerably in size and structure. Unless specifically stained, they are not visible. In addition to supplying cellular energy, mitochondria are involved in other tasks, such as cell signalling, cellular differentiation, and cell death, as well as maintaining control of the cell cycle and cell growth.

Modal logic

This is a type of formal logic which extends classical propositional and predicate logic to include operators expressing modality. A modal - a word that expresses a modality - qualifies a statement. For example, the statement "John is happy" might be qualified by saying that John is usually happy, in which case the term "usually" is functioning as a modal.

Monolithic architecture

Related to software, monolithic architecture is one in which functionally distinguishable aspects (for example data input and output, data processing, error handling, and the user interface) are all interwoven, rather than containing architecturally separate components.

Motion planning (also known as the navigation problem)

This is a term used in robotics for the process of breaking down a desired movement task into discrete motions that satisfy movement constraints and possibly optimize some aspect of the movement. Motion planning is the process of breaking down a movement task into "primitives" such as individual joint movements. Such movement often involves compliant motion, a process where movement requires maintaining physical contact with an object. Moravec's paradox generalizes that low-level sensorimotor skills that humans take for granted are, counterintuitively, difficult to program into a robot; the paradox is named after Hans Moravec, who stated in 1988 that "it is comparatively easy to make computers exhibit adult level performance on intelligence tests or playing checkers, and difficult or impossible to give them the skills of a one-year-old when it comes to perception and mobility". This is attributed to the fact that, unlike checkers, physical dexterity has been a direct target of natural selection for millions of years.

Multi-agent system (MAS or "self-organized system") is a computerized system composed of multiple interacting intelligent agents. Multi-agent systems can solve problems that are difficult or impossible for an individual agent or a monolithic system to solve.

Multimodal sentiment analysis

This is a new dimension of the traditional text-based sentiment analysis, which goes beyond the analysis of texts, and includes other modalities such as audio and visual data. It can be bimodal, which includes different combinations of two modalities, or trimodal, which incorporates three modalities. With the extensive amount of social media data available online in different forms such as videos and images, the conventional text-based sentiment analysis has evolved into more complex models of multimodal analysis of news videos, and emotion recognition (sometimes known as emotion detection) such as depression monitoring, among others.

Nany-valued logic (also multi- or multiple-valued logic) is a propositional calculus in which there are more than two truth values.

Natural language processing (NLP) gives machines the ability to read and understand human language. A sufficiently powerful natural language processing system would enable natural language user interfaces and the acquisition of knowledge directly from human-written sources, such as newswire texts. Some straightforward applications of natural language processing include information retrieval, text mining, question answering and machine translation. Many current approaches use word co-occurrence frequencies to construct syntactic representations of text. "Keyword spotting" strategies for search are popular and scalable but dumb: a search query for "dog" might only match documents with the literal word "dog" and miss a document with the word "poodle". "Lexical affinity" strategies use the occurrence of words such as "accident" to assess the sentiment of a document. Modern statistical NLP approaches can combine all these strategies as well as others, and often achieve acceptable accuracy at the page or paragraph level but continue to lack the semantic understanding required to classify isolated sentences well. Besides the usual difficulties with encoding semantic commonsense knowledge, existing semantic NLP sometimes scales too poorly to be viable in business applications. Beyond semantic NLP, the ultimate goal of "narrative" NLP is to embody a full understanding of commonsense reasoning.

Natural language understanding (NLU) or natural language interpretation (NLI)

This is a subtopic of natural language processing in artificial intelligence that deals with machine reading comprehension.

Natural-language user interfaces (NLUI)

These are a type of computer human interface where linguistic phenomena such as verbs, phrases and clauses act as user interface controls for creating, selecting and modifying data in software applications.

Neural network (NN)

This is an interconnected group of nodes, akin to the vast network of neurons in the human brain. Neural networks, or neural nets, were inspired by the architecture of neurons in the human brain. A simple "neuron" N accepts input from multiple other neurons, each of which, when activated (or "fired"), cast a weighted "vote" for or against whether neuron N should itself activate. Learning requires an algorithm to adjust these weights based on the training data. One simple algorithm (dubbed "fire together, wire together") is to increase the weight between two connected neurons when the activation of one triggers the successful activation of another. The net forms "concepts" that are distributed among a subnetwork of shared neurons that tend to fire together: a concept meaning "leg" might be coupled with a subnetwork meaning "foot" that includes the sound for "foot". Neurons have a continuous spectrum of activation; in addition, neurons can process inputs in a nonlinear way rather than weighing straightforward votes. Modern neural nets can learn both continuous functions and, surprisingly, digital logical operations. Neural networks' early successes included predicting the stock market and (in 1995) a mostly self-driving car. In the 2010s, advances in neural networks using deep learning thrust AI into widespread public consciousness and contributed to an enormous upshift in corporate AI spending; for example, AI-related company mergers and acquisitions in 2017 was over 25 times as large as in 2015.

Node

A node is an artificial neuron which makes up part of an artificial neural network.

Noise in AI

Humans are prone to making mistakes when collecting data, and data collection instruments may be unreliable, resulting in dataset errors. The errors are referred to as noise. Data noise in machine learning can cause problems since the algorithm interprets the noise as a pattern and can start generalizing from it.

Non-monotonic logic is a formal logic whose consequence relation is not monotonic. In other words, non-monotonic logics are devised to capture and represent defeasible inferences, i.e., a kind of inference in which reasoners draw tentative conclusions, enabling reasoners to retract their conclusion(s) based on further evidence.

Nouvelle AI differs from classical AI by aiming to produce robots with intelligence levels similar to insects. Researchers believe that intelligence can emerge organically from simple behaviours as these intelligences interacted with the "real world," instead of using the constructed worlds which symbolic AIs typically needed to have programmed into them.

Nucleus

This is a membrane-enclosed organelle found in eukaryotic cells.

Occam's razor

This is the problem-solving principle that the simplest solution tends to be the right one. When presented with competing hypotheses to solve a problem, one should select the solution with the fewest assumptions. The idea is attributed to William of Ockham (c. 1287–1347), who was an English Franciscan friar, scholastic philosopher, and theologian. In science, Occam's razor is used as an abductive heuristic in the development of theoretical models, rather than as a rigorous arbiter between candidate models.

Opinion mining

Opinion mining (sometimes known as sentiment analysis or emotion AI) refers to the use of natural language processing, text analysis, computational linguistics, and biometrics to systematically identify, extract, quantify, and study affective states and subjective information. Sentiment analysis is widely applied to voice of the customer materials such as reviews and survey responses, online and social media, and healthcare materials for applications that range from marketing to customer service to clinical medicine.

Optical character recognition (OCR)

Optical character recognition is the mechanical or electronic conversion of images of typed, handwritten or printed text into machine-encoded text, whether from a scanned document, a photo of a document, a scene-photo (for example the text on signs and billboards in a landscape photo) or from subtitle text superimposed on an image

Optimization

In mathematics, computer science and operations research, optimization is the selection of a best element (with regard to a specific criterion) from some set of available alternatives. For many problems, it is possible to begin the search with some form of a guess and then refine the guess incrementally until no more refinements can be made. These algorithms can be visualized as blind hill climbing: the search is initiated at a random point on the landscape, and then, by jumps or steps, it keeps moving the guess uphill, until the top is reached. Other optimization algorithms are simulated annealing, beam search and random optimization.

P versus NP

The general class of questions for which some algorithm can provide an answer in polynomial time is called "class P" or just "P". For some questions, there is no known way to find an answer quickly, but if one is provided with information showing what the answer is, it is possible to verify the answer quickly. The class of questions for which an answer can be verified in polynomial time is called NP, which stands for "nondeterministic polynomial time. The P versus NP problem is a major unsolved problem in computer science. It asks whether every problem whose solution can be quickly verified (technically, verified in polynomial time) can also be solved quickly (again, in polynomial time).

Partial derivative of a function of several variables

This is the derivative with respect to one of those variables, with the others held constant (as opposed to the total derivative, in which all variables are allowed to vary).

Pattern recognition is a branch of machine learning that focuses on the recognition of patterns and regularities in data, although it is in some cases considered to be nearly synonymous with machine learning

Perceptron

This is a learning network with a single layer, similar to the old concept of linear regression. The main categories of networks are acyclic or feedforward neural networks (where the signal passes in only one direction) and recurrent neural networks (which allow feedback and short-term memories of previous input events). Among the most popular feedforward networks are perceptrons, multi-layer perceptrons and radial basis networks. Neural networks can be applied to the problem of intelligent control (for robotics) or learning, using such techniques as Hebbian learning ("fire together, wire together"), GMDH or competitive learning. Today, neural networks are often trained by the backpropagation algorithm.

Pheromone (see ant colony organization)

Pheromones are chemical signals, that is, carriers of information between individuals within a species. Pheromones induce a physiological or behavioural response in the receiving individual, and often play a crucial role in mate finding and other interactions among animals.

Pixel

In digital imaging a pixel is the smallest addressable element in a raster image, or the smallest addressable element in a dot matrix display device. In most digital display devices, pixels are the smallest element that can be manipulated through software. In computer graphics and digital photography, a raster image represents a two-dimensional picture as a rectangular matrix or grid of square pixels, viewable via a computer display, paper, or other display medium. A raster is technically characterized by the width and height of the image in pixels and by the number of bits per pixel. Each pixel is a sample of an original or synthetic image; more samples typically provide more accurate representations of the original. The intensity of each pixel is variable. In color imaging systems, a color is typically represented by three or four component intensities such as red, green, and blue, or cyan, magenta, yellow, and black.

Predictive analytics

This encompasses a variety of statistical techniques from data mining, predictive modelling, and machine learning, that analyze current and historical facts to make predictions about future or otherwise unknown events

Probabilistic logic (also probability logic and probabilistic reasoning) is the combination of capacity of probability theory to handle uncertainty and the capacity of deductive logic to exploit structure of formal argument. The result is a richer and more expressive formalism with a broad range of possible application areas. Probabilistic logics attempt to find a natural extension of traditional logic truth tables: the results they define are derived through probabilistic expressions.

Probability

This measure is a real-valued function defined on a set of events in a probability space that satisfies measure properties such as countable additivity. The difference between a probability measure and the more general notion of measure (which includes concepts like area or volume) is that a probability measure must assign value 1 to the entire probability space.

Probability space

This is a mathematical construct that models a real-world process (or "experiment") consisting of states that occur randomly. A probability space is constructed with a specific kind of situation or experiment in mind. It proposes that each time a situation of that kind arises, the set of possible outcomes is the same and the probabilities are also the same.

Probability theory is the branch of mathematics concerned with probability. Although there are several different probability interpretations, probability theory treats the concept in a rigorous mathematical manner by expressing it through a set of axioms. Typically these axioms formalise probability in terms of a probability space, which assigns a measure taking values between 0 and 1, termed the probability measure, to a set of outcomes called the sample space. Any specified subset of these outcomes is called an event. The first axiom of probability theory is a non-negative real number.

Probability is the measure of the likelihood that an event will occur.

Processor or processing units

These are electronic circuits which performs operations on some external data source, usually memory or some other data stream.

Prokaryotes

These are unicellular organism that lacks a membrane-bound nucleus, mitochondria, or any other membrane-bound organelle. Bacteria and algae are examples.

Propositional calculus

This is a branch of logic and is also called propositional logic, statement logic, sentential calculus, or sentential logic. It deals with propositions (which can be true or false) and argument flow. Compound propositions are formed by connecting propositions by logical connectives. The propositions without logical connectives are called atomic propositions. Unlike first-order logic, propositional logic does not deal with non-logical objects, predicates about them, or quantifiers. However, all the machinery of propositional logic is included in first-order logic and higher-order logics. In this sense, propositional logic is the foundation of first-order logic and higher-order logic.

Propositional logic

This is also known as statement logic, sentential calculus, or sentential logic. It deals with propositions (which can be true or false). Propositional calculus is a branch of logic. It deals with propositions (which can be true or false) and argument flow. Several different forms of logic are used in AI research. Propositional logic involves truth functions such as "or" and "not". Several extensions of logic have been designed to handle specific domains of knowledge, such as description logics, situation calculus, event calculus and fluent calculus (for representing events and time), causal calculus, belief calculus and modal logics.

Qualification problem

In philosophy and AI (especially in knowledge-based systems) this is concerned with the impossibility of listing all the preconditions required for a real-world action to have its intended effect. It might be posed as how to deal with the things that prevent the achievement of an intended result. It is strongly connected to, and opposite the ramification side of, the frame problem.

Radial basis function (RBF)

This is a real-valued function whose value depends only on the distance from the origin. A radial basis function network is an artificial neural network that uses radial basis functions as activation functions. The output of the network is a linear combination of radial basis functions of the inputs and neuron parameters. Radial basis function networks have many uses, including function approximation, time series prediction, classification, and system control.

Random forest or random decision forests

This is an ensemble learning method for classification, regression and other tasks that operates by constructing a multitude of decision trees at training time. For classification tasks, the output of the random forest is the class selected by most trees. For regression tasks, the mean or average prediction of the individual trees is returned.

Random optimization (RO)

This is a family of numerical optimization methods that do not require the gradient of the problem to be optimized and RO can hence be used on functions that are not continuous or differentiable. Such optimization methods are also known as direct-search, derivative-free, or black-box methods.

Random variables, (also known as random quantities, aleatory variables, or stochastic variables)

These are variables whose possible values are outcomes of a random phenomenon. As a function, a random variable is required to be measurable, which rules out certain pathological cases where the quantity which the random variable returns is infinitely sensitive to small changes in the outcome. Random variables have a lack of pattern or predictability in events.

Rational choice theory

Also known as choice theory or rational action theory, this is a framework for understanding, and often formally modelling, social and economic behaviour. The basic premise of rational choice theory is that aggregate social behaviour results from the behaviour of individual actors, each of whom is making their individual decisions. The theory also focuses on the determinants of the individual choices (methodological individualism).

Reasoning

This was an early approach to searching using developed algorithms that imitated step-by-step the reasoning that humans use when they solve puzzles or make logical deductions. Simple exhaustive searches are rarely sufficient for most real-world problems: the search space (the number of places to search) quickly grows to astronomical numbers. The result is a search that is too slow or that never completes. The solution, for many problems, is to use heuristics or "rules of thumb" that prioritize choices in favour of those that are more likely to reach a goal and to do so in a shorter number of steps. In some search methodologies heuristics can also serve to entirely eliminate some choices that are unlikely to lead to a goal (called "pruning the search tree"). Heuristics supply the program with a "best guess" for the path on which the solution lies. Heuristics limit the search for solutions into a smaller sample size.

Recurrent neural network (RNN)

This is a class of artificial neural network where connections between nodes form a directed graph along a sequence. This allows it to exhibit temporal dynamic behaviour for a time sequence. Unlike feedforward neural networks, RNNs can use their internal state (memory) to process sequences of inputs. This makes them applicable to tasks such as unsegmented, connected handwriting recognition or speech recognition.

*Reinforcement learnin*g (RL)

Reinforcement learning is concerned with how an agent ought to take actions in an environment so as to maximize some notion of long-term reward. Reinforcement learning algorithms attempt to find a policy that maps states of the world to the actions the agent ought to take in those states. Reinforcement learning differs from the supervised learning problem in that correct input/output pairs are never presented, nor sub-optimal actions explicitly corrected. Training data (in the form of rewards and punishments) is given only as feedback to the program's actions in a dynamic environment, such as driving a vehicle or playing a game against an opponent.

Representation learning

Researchers at the Massachusetts Institute of Technology (MIT) found that solving difficult problems in vision and natural language processing required ad-hoc solutions – they argued that there was no simple and general principle (like logic) that would capture all the aspects of intelligent behavior. Roger Schank described their "anti-logic" approaches as "scruffy" (as opposed to the "neat" paradigms used at universities such as Carnegie Mellon and Stanford Universities). Commonsense knowledge bases are an example of "scruffy" AI, since they must be built by hand, one complicated concept at a time. Representation learning algorithms often attempt to preserve the information in their input but transform it in a way that makes it useful, often as a pre-processing step before performing classification or predictions, allowing reconstruction of the inputs coming from the unknown data generating distribution, while not being necessarily faithful for configurations that are implausible under that distribution.

Restricted Boltzmann machine (RBM) is a generative stochastic artificial neural network that can learn a probability distribution over its set of inputs.

Robotics

This is an interdisciplinary branch of engineering and science that includes mechanical engineering, electronics engineering, computer science, and others. Robotics deals with the design, construction, operation, and use of robots, as well as computer systems for their control, sensory feedback, and information processing. AI is heavily used in robotics. Advanced robotic arms and other industrial robots, widely used in modern factories, can learn from experience how to move efficiently despite the presence of friction and gear slippage. A modern mobile robot, when given a small, static, and visible environment, can easily determine its location and map its environment; however, dynamic environments, such as in endoscopy (examining the interior of a patient's breathing body) pose a greater challenge. Robots can be guided by an external control device or the control may be embedded within. Robots may be constructed to take on human form but most robots are machines designed to perform a task with no regard as to how they look.

Rule of inference

Also known as inference rule or transformation rule), rule of inference is a logical form consisting of a function which takes premises, analyzes their syntax, and returns a conclusion (or conclusions).

Rule-based machine learning

Rule-based systems are used as a way to store and manipulate knowledge to interpret information in a useful way. They are often used in artificial intelligence applications and research.

Sample space

In probability theory of an experiment or random trial this is the set of all possible outcomes or results of that experiment.

Satplan

(Better known as Planning as Satisfiability), this is a method for automated planning. It converts the planning problem instance into an instance of the Boolean satisfiability problem, which is then solved using a method for establishing satisfiability such as the DPLL algorithm or WalkSAT.

Search and optimization

Many problems in AI can be solved in theory by intelligently searching through many possible solutions: Reasoning can be reduced to performing a search. For example, logical proof can be viewed as searching for a path that leads from premises to conclusions, where each step is the application of an inference rule. Planning algorithms search through trees of goals and subgoals, attempting to find a path to a target goal, a process called means-ends analysis. Robotics algorithms for moving limbs and grasping objects use local searches in configuration space. Many learning algorithms use search algorithms based on optimization.

Semi-supervised learning

The computer is given only an incomplete training signal: a training set with some (often many) of the target outputs missing.

Sequence learning

In cognitive psychology, this is inherent to human ability because it is an integrated part of conscious and nonconscious learning as well as activities. Sequences of information or sequences of actions are used in various everyday tasks: from sequencing sounds in speech, to sequencing movements in typing or playing instruments, to sequencing actions in driving an automobile. Sequence learning can be used to study skill acquisition and in studies of various groups. According to Ritter and Nerb, “The order in which material is presented can strongly influence what is learned, how fast performance increases, and sometimes even whether the material is learned at all.” Sequence learning, more known and understood as a form of explicit learning, is now also being studied as a form of implicit learning as well as other forms of learning. Sequence learning can also be referred to as sequential behaviour, behaviour sequencing, and serial order in behavior.

Set theory

This is a branch of mathematical logic that studies sets, which informally are collections of objects. Although any type of object can be collected into a set, set theory is applied most often to objects that are relevant to mathematics. The language of set theory can be used in the definitions of nearly all mathematical objects.

Similarity and metric learning

Similarity learning is closely related to distance metric learning. Metric learning is the task of learning a distance function over objects. A metric or distance function has to obey four axioms: non-negativity, identity of indiscernibles, symmetry and subadditivity (or the triangle inequality).

Simulated annealing (SA)

This is a probabilistic technique for approximating the global optimum of a given function. Specifically, it is a metaheuristic to approximate global optimization in a large search space. It is often used when the search space is discrete (e.g., all tours that visit a given set of cities). For problems where finding an approximate global optimum is more important than finding a precise local optimum in a fixed amount of time, simulated annealing may be preferable to alternatives such as gradient descent.

Situated agents

These are agents which are embedded in an environment. The term situated is commonly used to refer to robots, but some researchers argue that software agents can also be situated.

Situation calculus

This represents changing scenarios as a set of first-order logic formulae. It is a logic formalism designed for representing and reasoning about dynamical domains.

SOAR is a cognitive architecture, originally created by John Laird, Allen Newell, and Paul Rosenbloom at Carnegie Mellon University. The goal of the SOAR project is to develop the fixed computational building blocks necessary for general intelligent agents – agents that can perform a wide range of tasks and encode, use, and learn all types of knowledge to realize the full range of cognitive capabilities found in humans, such as decision making, problem solving, planning, and natural language understanding. It is both a theory of what cognition is and a computational implementation of that theory.

Social intelligence (also known as Affective computing)

This is an interdisciplinary umbrella that comprises systems which recognize, interpret, process, or simulate human affects. Moderate successes related to affective computing include textual sentiment analysis and, more recently, multimodal affect analysis, in which AI classifies the affects displayed by a videotaped subject. In the long run, social skills and an understanding of human emotion and game theory would be valuable to a social agent. Being able to predict the actions of others by understanding their motives and emotional states would allow an agent to make better decisions. Some computer systems mimic human emotion and expressions to appear more sensitive to the emotional dynamics of human interaction, or to otherwise facilitate human - computer interaction. Similarly, some virtual assistants are programmed to speak conversationally or even to banter humorously; this tends to give naive users an unrealistic conception of how intelligent existing computer agents actually are. Social intelligence comprises social skills and an understanding of human emotion and game theory. Some computer systems mimic human emotion and expressions to appear more sensitive to the emotional dynamics of human interaction, or to otherwise facilitate human–computer interaction.

Soft Computing (SC)

This has as its principal constituents Fuzzy Logic, Evolutionary Computation, Machine Learning and Probabilistic Reasoning, with the latter subsuming belief networks and parts of learning theory. Soft computing (sometimes referred to as computational intelligence, is the use of inexact solutions to computationally hard tasks, for which there is no known algorithm that can compute an exact solution in polynomial time. Soft computing differs from conventional (hard) computing in that, unlike hard computing, it is tolerant of imprecision, uncertainty, partial truth, and approximation. In effect, the role model for soft computing is the human mind.

AI planning

Sometimes denoted as AI Planning, automated planning and scheduling is a branch of artificial intelligence that concerns the realization of strategies or action sequences, typically for execution by intelligent agents, autonomous robots and unmanned vehicles. Unlike classical control and classification problems, the solutions are complex and must be discovered and optimized in a multidimensional space.

Sparse dictionary learning

Statistical learning in AI is the adoption of sophisticated mathematical tools, such as hidden Markov models, information theory, and normative Bayesian decision theory to compare or to unify competing architectures. The shared mathematical language permits a high level of collaboration with more established fields (like mathematics, economics or operations research).

Stochastic neural network

This is a type of artificial neural networks built by introducing random variations into the network, either by giving the network's neurons stochastic transfer functions, or by giving them stochastic weights. This makes them useful tools for optimization problems, since the random fluctuations help it escape from local minima. An example of a neural network using stochastic transfer functions is a Boltzmann machine. Each neuron is binary valued, and the chance of it firing depends on the other neurons in the network. Stochastic neural networks have found applications in risk management, oncology, bioinformatics, and other similar fields.

Stochastic optimization (SO) methods

These are optimization methods that generate and use random variables. For stochastic problems, the random variables appear in the formulation of the optimization problem itself, which involve random objective functions or random constraints. Stochastic optimization methods also include methods with random iterates. Some stochastic optimization methods use random iterates to solve stochastic problems, combining both meanings of stochastic optimization. Stochastic optimization methods generalize deterministic methods for deterministic problems. Stochastic optimization methods are optimization methods that generate and use random variables. For stochastic problems, the random variables appear in the formulation of the optimization problem itself, which involve random objective functions or random constraints. Stochastic optimization methods also include methods with random iterates.

Stochastic

This is an adjective that describes something that was randomly determined.

Sub-symbolic AI

By the 1980s progress in symbolic AI seemed to stall and many believed that symbolic systems would never be able to imitate all the processes of human cognition, especially perception, robotics, learning and pattern recognition. A number of researchers began to look into "sub-symbolic" approaches to specific AI problems. Sub-symbolic methods manage to approach intelligence without specific representations of knowledge.

Supervised learning

The computer is presented with example inputs and their desired outputs, given by a "teacher", and the goal is to learn a general rule that maps inputs to outputs; the input signal can be only partially available, or restricted to special feedback.

Supervised learning

The computer is presented with example inputs and their desired outputs, given by a "teacher", and the goal is to learn a general rule that maps inputs to outputs; the input signal can be only partially available, or restricted to special feedback:

Support vector machines

Support vector machines (SVMs) are a set of related supervised learning methods used for classification and regression. Given a set of training examples, each marked as belonging to one of two categories, an SVM training algorithm builds a model that predicts whether a new example falls into one category or the other. Support vector machines, also known as support vector networks in machine learning, are supervised learning models with associated learning algorithms that analyse data used for classification and regression analysis. Given a set of training examples, each marked as belonging to one or the other of two categories, an SVM training algorithm builds a model that assigns new examples to one category or the other, making it a non-probabilistic binary linear classifier.

Swarm intelligence (SI)

This is the collective behaviour of decentralized, natural or artificial self-organized systems. SI systems consist typically of a population of simple agents or boids interacting locally with one another and with their environment. The inspiration often comes from nature, especially biological systems. The agents follow very simple rules, and although there is no centralized control structure dictating how individual agents should behave, local, and to a certain degree random, interactions between such agents lead to the emergence of "intelligent" global behavior, unknown to the individual agents. Examples in natural systems of SI include ant colonies, bird flocking, animal herding, bacterial growth, fish schooling and microbial intelligence.

Symbolic AI

When access to digital computers became possible in the middle 1950s, AI research began to explore the possibility that human intelligence could be reduced to symbol manipulation. The research was centered in three institutions: Carnegie Mellon University, Stanford and the Massachusetts Institute of Technology (MIT), and each one developed its own style of research. John Haugeland named these symbolic approaches to AI "good old fashioned AI" or "GOFAI". During the 1960s symbolic approaches had achieved great success at simulating high-level thinking in small demonstration programs. Approaches based on cybernetics or artificial neural networks were abandoned or pushed into the background. Symbolic artificial intelligence is the term for the collection of all methods in artificial intelligence research that are based on high-level "symbolic" (human-readable) representations of problems, logic and search. Symbolic AI was the dominant paradigm of AI research from the mid-1950s until the late 1980s.

Syntax

This is anything having to do with formal languages or formal systems without regard to any interpretation or meaning given to them. Syntax is concerned with the rules used for constructing, or transforming the symbols and words of a language, as contrasted with the semantics of a language which are concerned with its meaning.

Sparse coding algorithms

These represent an attempt to work under the constraint that the learned representation is low-dimensional. They attempt to do so under the constraint that the learned representation is sparse (ie has many zeros). Multilinear subspace learning algorithms aim to learn low-dimensional representations directly from tensor representations for multidimensional data, without reshaping them into high-dimensional vectors.

Transfer learning

Transfer learning is a research problem in machine learning that focuses on storing knowledge gained while solving one problem and applying it to a different but related problem. For example, knowledge gained while learning to recognize cars could apply when trying to recognize trucks.

Transformer

Transformer is a deep learning architecture based on the multi-head attention mechanism. It is notable for not containing any recurrent units, and thus requires less training time than previous recurrent neural architectures.

Truth value

This is sometimes called a logical value, in logic and mathematics, and is a value indicating the relationship of a proposition to truth.

U-net

U-Net architecture stems from the so-called “fully convolutional network”. The main idea is to supplement a usual contracting network by successive layers, where pooling operations are replaced by upsampling operators. In contrast, with CNN the image is converted into a vector which is largely used in classification problems. In U-Net an image is converted into a vector and then the same mapping is used to convert it again to an image. This reduces the distortion by preserving the original structure of the image.

Unstructured data (or unstructured information)

This is information that either does not have a pre-defined data model or is not organized in a pre-defined manner. Unstructured information is typically text-heavy, but may contain data such as dates, numbers, and facts as well. This results in irregularities and ambiguities that make it difficult to understand using traditional programs as compared to data stored in fielded form in databases or annotated (semantically tagged) in documents.

Unsupervised learning

This is a machine learning task of inferring a function that describes the structure of "unlabelled" data (i.e. data that have not been classified or categorized). Since the examples given to the learning algorithm are unlabelled, there is no straightforward way to evaluate the accuracy of the structure that is produced by the algorithm - one feature that distinguishes unsupervised learning from supervised learning and reinforcement learning. No labels are given to the learning algorithm, leaving it on its own to find structure in its input. Unsupervised learning can be a goal in itself (discovering hidden patterns in data) or a means towards an end (feature learning)

Vanishing gradient problem

This is a difficulty found in training artificial neural networks with gradient-based learning methods and backpropagation. In such methods, each of the neural network's weights receives an update proportional to the partial derivative of the error function with respect to the current weight in each iteration of training. The problem is that in some cases, the gradient will be vanishingly small, effectively preventing the weight from changing its value. In the worst case, this may completely stop the neural network from further training.

Waggle dance

This is a term used in beekeeping and ethology for a particular figure-eight dance of the honey bee. By performing this dance, successful foragers can share, with other members of the colony, information about the direction and distance to patches of flowers yielding nectar and pollen, to water sources, or to new nest-site locations.

WalkSAT (and *GSAT)* are local search algorithms to solve Boolean satisfiability problems. Both algorithms work on formulae in Boolean logic that are in, or have been converted into, conjunctive normal form. They start by assigning a random value to each variable in the formula. If the assignment satisfies all clauses, the algorithm terminates, returning the assignment. Otherwise, a variable is flipped and the above is then repeated until all the clauses are satisfied.

Zero-sum game

In game theory and economic theory a zero-sum game is a mathematical representation of a situation in which each participant's gain or loss of utility is exactly balanced by the losses or gains of the utility of the other participants. If the total gains of the participants are added up and the total losses are subtracted, they will sum to zero.

Chapter 2. An introduction to artificial intelligence and machine learning

Introduction

Artificial intelligence (AI) is the use of data to solve complex problems.

It involves the use of machines (ie computers) that can learn by themselves, rather than being taught (programmed) by humans to perform tasks normally requiring human intelligence, such as visual perception, speech recognition, decision-making, and translation between languages. In simple terms AI is the capability of a machine to imitate intelligent human behaviour. AI is comprised of a number of algorithms and computer code. AI involves logic and data input, all resulting in data output.

What is an algorithm?

A programming algorithm can be thought of as a recipe that describes the exact steps needed for the computer to solve a problem or reach a goal. An algorithm can be compared to a food recipe with a list of the ingredients needed and a set of steps on how to make the intended meal. In computer terms, the word for a recipe is a procedure, and the ingredients are called inputs. A programming algorithm describes what the computer should do, and the computer will do it exactly that way every time. The process of folding a shirt or a pair of trousers is an algorithm, as are the activities people do when they wake up: these would be the inputs for the latter:

Wake up

Take shower

Do exercises

Have breakfast

Dress for work

Wait for transport to work

The output would be “Typical activities early on a weekday morning”.

Another simple example of an algorithm would be to find the largest number in an unsorted list of numbers. If there was a list of five different numbers, this can be easily done without the help of a computer, but if there are five million different numbers a computer will be required, and a computer needs an algorithm. This is what the algorithm could look like: the input consists of a list of numbers, and this list is called L. The number L1 would be the first number in the list, L2 the second number, and so on. Thus, the input to the algorithm is a list of numbers, and the output would be the largest number in the list.

Algorithms can perform calculations, data processing and automated reasoning tasks.

Another way to describe an algorithm is a sequence of unambiguous instructions. A procedure for solving a mathematical problem (such as finding the highest common factor) is a finite number of steps in a step-by-step procedure. An algorithm can be expressed within a finite amount of space and time and in a well-defined formal language for calculating a function. Starting from an initial state and initial input, the instructions describe a computation that, when executed, proceeds through a finite number of well-defined successive states, eventually producing an output. The transition from one state to the next is not necessarily deterministic; some algorithms, known as randomized algorithms, incorporate random input.

It is important, however, to note that a programming algorithm is not computer code. It can be written in everyday language. It has a start, a middle, and an end. It includes only what is needed to carry out the task. It does not include anything that is unclear or ambiguous. Although algorithms can be written in regular language, it takes a long time to do so. Therefore, algorithms are now usually written in programming languages such as Cobal, Fortran or Python.

The traditional algorithmic approach to image analysis for classification previously relied on (1) handcrafted object segmentation, followed by (2) identification of each segmented object using statistical classifiers or shallow neural computational machine-learning classifiers designed specifically for each class of objects, and finally (3) classification of the image. Creating and refining multiple classifiers required many skilled people and much time and was computationally expensive.

The development of convolutional neural network layers has allowed for significant gains in the ability to classify images and detect objects in a picture

These are multiple processing layers to which image analysis filters, or convolutions, are applied. The abstracted representation of images within each layer is constructed by systematically convolving multiple filters across the image, producing a feature map that is used as input to the following layer. This architecture makes it possible to process images in the form of pixels as input and to give the desired classification as output. The image-to-classification approach in one classifier replaces the multiple steps of previous image analysis methods.

One method of addressing a lack of data in a given domain is to leverage data from a similar domain, a technique known as transfer learning. Transfer learning has proven to be a highly effective technique, particularly when faced with domains with limited data.

Rather than training a completely blank network, by using a feed-forward approach to fix the weights in the lower levels already optimized to recognize the structures found in images in general and retraining the weights of the upper levels with back propagation, the model can recognize the distinguishing features of a specific category of images, such as images of the eye, much faster and with significantly fewer training examples and less computational power

Computer programming

Computer programming or coding is the composition of sequences of instructions, called programs, that computers follow to perform tasks. It involves designing and implementing algorithms, step-by-step specifications of procedures, by writing code in one or more programming languages. Programmers typically use high-level programming languages that are more easily intelligible to humans than machine code, which is directly executed by the central processing unit of the computer. Proficient programming usually requires expertise in several different subjects, including knowledge of the application domain, details of programming languages and generic code libraries, specialized algorithms, and formal logic.

What is computer code?

Source code, or simply code, is any collection of text written using a human-readable programming language, usually as plain text. The source code of a program is specially designed to facilitate the work of computer programmers, who specify the actions to be performed by a computer mostly by writing source code.

Source code is the version of software as it is originally written (i.e., typed into a computer) by a human in plain text (i.e., human readable alphanumeric characters).

How do machines learn?

In one of two ways:

1. by having their incorrect outputs revised by human input

This is straightforward: for example, if 10,000 images of a melanoma are uploaded into the computer's memory labelled as "melanoma" and then 10,000 images of a benign freckle labelled as "benign freckle" are uploaded, a photograph of a dark skin lesion can then be uploaded and the computer can be asked to diagnose it as either "melanoma" or "benign freckle". If it gets the diagnosis incorrectly, this can be corrected and the computer's learning ability is thereby increased and improved.

2. by insertion of a length of computer code

This is more difficult but useful: insertion of a length of computer code picks up errors in output and automatically improves the computer's output ability.

Computers are learning how to code themselves

Snyk is a company focused on an all-in-one platform for securing computer code. Snyk's DeepCoder is a machine learning system that can write its own code. It does this using a technique called program synthesis. Essentially, it creates new programs by combining existing lines of code taken from other software, which is what human coders do. With a particular output in mind, DeepCoder is able to determine which lines or pieces of code are likely to be particularly useful. The approach is to train a neural network to predict properties of the program that generated the outputs from the inputs. DeepCoder can trawl through the basic, input-output style challenges usually set by programming competitions. It is able to search through lines of code more thoroughly and widely than a human coder could, quickly piecing together code in a manner humans might not think of. Because DeepCoder is essentially a deep learning algorithm, every time it is given a new problem, it gets better at combining lines from source codes. Ultimately, this algorithm can make programming accessible to non-coders, allowing anyone to easily build simple programs. DeepCoder's current version only allows it to handle programming challenges with around five lines of code. Future versions of DeepCode may facilitate building routine programs that take information from websites without the need for human coders.

Modifying/Improving programs

It is now possible for a computer program to write its own programs.

Types of artificial intelligence

AI can be categorized in any number of ways; here are two examples. The first classifies AI systems as either weak AI or strong AI. Weak AI, also known as narrow AI, is an AI system that is designed and trained for a particular task. Virtual personal assistants, such as Apple's Siri, are a form of weak AI. Strong AI, also known as artificial general intelligence, is an AI system with generalized human cognitive abilities so that when presented with an unfamiliar task, it has enough intelligence to find a solution.

Arend Hintze categorized AI into four types, from the kind of AI systems that exist today to sentient systems, which do not yet exist. His categories are as follows:

Type 1: Reactive machines. An example is Deep Blue, the IBM chess program that beat Garry Kasparov in the 1990s. Deep Blue can identify pieces on the chess board and make predictions, but it has no memory and cannot use past experiences to inform future ones. It analyzes possible moves - its own and those of its opponent - and chooses the most strategic move. Deep Blue and Google's AlphaGo were designed for narrow purposes and cannot easily be applied to other situations.

Type 2: Limited memory. These AI systems can use past experiences to inform future decisions. Some of the decision-making functions in autonomous vehicles have been designed this way. Observations can be used to inform actions such as a car that has changed lanes. These observations are not stored permanently.

Type 3: Theory of mind. This is a psychology term. It refers to the understanding that others have their own beliefs, desires and intentions that impact the decisions they make. This kind of AI does not yet exist.

Type 4: Self-awareness. In this category, AI systems have a sense of self and consciousness. Machines with self-awareness understand their current state and can use the information to infer what others are feeling. This type of AI does not yet exist.

Examples of AI technology

Automation is the process of making a system or process function automatically. Robotic process automation (RPA), for example, can be programmed to perform high-volume, repeatable tasks normally performed by humans. RPA is different from IT automation in that it can adapt to changing circumstances.

There are three types of machine learning algorithms

Supervised learning, in which data sets are labelled so that patterns can be detected and used to label new data sets; unsupervised learning, in which data sets are not labelled and are sorted according to similarities or differences; and reinforcement learning, in which data sets are not labelled but, after performing an action or several actions, the AI system is given feedback.

Machine vision

Machine vision is the science of making computers see. Machine vision captures and analyzes visual information using a camera, analog-to-digital conversion and digital signal processing. It is often compared to human eyesight, but machine vision is not bound by biology and can be programmed to see through walls, for example. It is used in a range of applications from signature identification to medical image analysis. There are four key tasks required of the computer. They are

1. image classification – assigning labels to the images, for example, liver metastases

2. object detection - locating and outlining specific entities on the image

3. semantic segmentation - assigning object category to each pixel in the image

4. instance segmentation - segmenting and labelling individual objects at the pixel level

Object recognition (also called object classification)

One or several pre-specified or learned objects or object classes can be recognized, usually together with their 2D positions in the image or 3D poses in the scene.

Identification

An individual instance of an object is recognized. Examples include identification of a specific person's face or fingerprint, identification of handwritten digits, or identification of a specific vehicle.

Detection

The image data are scanned for specific objects along with their locations. Examples include the detection of an obstacle in the car's field of view and possible abnormal cells or tissues in medical images or the detection of a vehicle in an automatic road toll system. Detection based on relatively simple and fast computations is sometimes used for finding smaller regions of interesting image data which can be further analyzed by more computationally demanding techniques to produce a correct interpretation.

Natural language processing (NLP)

This is the processing of human - and not computer - language by a computer program. One of the older and best-known examples of NLP is spam detection, which looks at the subject line and the text of an email and decides if it is spam. Current approaches to NLP are based on machine learning. NLP tasks include text translation, sentiment analysis and speech recognition.

Pattern recognition

This is a branch of machine learning that focuses on identifying patterns in data.

Robotics is a field of engineering focused on the design and manufacturing of robots. Robots are often used to perform tasks that are difficult for humans to perform or perform consistently. They are used in assembly lines for car production or by NASA to move large objects in space. More recently, researchers are using machine learning to build robots that can interact in social settings.

Improving patient outcomes and reducing costs

Companies are applying machine learning to make better and faster diagnoses than humans. One of the best-known healthcare technologies is IBM Watson. IBM Watson is designed for a wide range of uses, including data analysis, healthcare, finance, and customer service. It understands natural language and is capable of responding to questions asked of it. The system mines patient data and other available data sources to form a hypothesis, which it then presents with a confidence scoring schema. In contrast, ChatGPT-4 is primarily designed for natural language processing tasks, such as chatbots, language translation, and text generation. In 2022 IBM divested and spun-off their Watson Health division into Merative. As of 2023, it remains a standalone company headquartered in Ann Arbor, Michigan.

Chatbots

Other AI applications include chatbots, a computer program used online to answer questions and assist customers, to help schedule follow-up appointments or aiding patients through the billing process, and virtual health assistants that provide basic medical feedback.

Current status of AI

In 2012 a series of experiments showed that neural networks fuelled with large sets of data and powerful computer chips gave machines new powers of perception. Deep learning, the rocket fuel of the current AI boom, is a revival of one of the oldest ideas in AI. The technique involves passing data through webs of mathematics loosely inspired by how brain cells work (known as artificial neural networks). As the network processes training data, connections between the parts of the network adjust, building up an ability to interpret future data.

Multimodal generative AI

The dream of precision health is to develop a continuous learning health system where new health information is instantly incorporated to optimize care delivery and accelerate biomedical discovery. Multimodal generative AI has the potential to drastically accelerate progress toward precision health by supercharging the structuring of health data and scaling population-level insight generation. Health data is inherently multimodal and longitudinal, comprising physical measurements and natural-language narratives. Only a fraction of such data is available in structured forms, as manual curation is costly and hard to scale. Multimodal generative AI can alleviate the curation bottleneck by leveraging self-supervision from cross-modal correspondence and help extract predictive signals not available in standalone modalities (Poon, 2024).

Modern generative AI takes self-supervision to the web scale, thus acquiring emergent capabilities not seen in smaller scale of pretraining. In a truly generalist fashion, large language models (LLMs) such as GPT-4 have demonstrated unprecedented prowess in conversation, reasoning, and instruction-following for new tasks without specialized training.

In health applications GPT-4 has already demonstrated its potentially transformative power from drafting in-basket responses to automating clinical documentation, and from scaling clinical trial matching to analyzing population-level real-world data (Fernandes et al., 2023). However, to fulfill the potential of generative AI in precision health, there are still big challenges, especially as the scope of multimodal data such as medical imaging and multi-omics is broadened.

Scaling Benchmark Creation and Evaluation

Perhaps counterintuitively, the most fundamental challenge facing health generative AI lies less in model building, but in creating realistic benchmarks that reflect real-world use cases, as well as scaling evaluation for complex generation tasks. Without reliable goalposts, it is hard to measure progress, especially for modern foundation models with open-ended capabilities, such as GPT-4V.

It is exciting to see a plethora of medical AI explorations in diagnostics. However, the potential impact of health generative AI is much broader, encompassing many low-risk yet high-value scenarios across the entire health system, from clerical and documentation tasks in health delivery, to clinical trials and post-market surveillance in drug development, to early biomedical discovery and value-based care.

To sustain and accelerate progress in health generative AI, it is thus necessary to invest in comprehensive benchmark creation and evaluation that represent diverse populations and real-world scenarios. Manual effort is not scalable, especially for accurate evaluation. Interestingly, generative AI itself may be harnessed to address this challenge. Powerful LLMs such as GPT-4 have already demonstrated remarkable capabilities in self-verifying its own output. It may seem paradoxical at first sight, but verification is often easier than generation, akin to P vs NP in computer science. Developing self-improving LLM-based agent systems to supercharge domain experts in benchmark creation and evaluation represents a key direction forward for health generative AI.

Bridging the health competency gap in large multimodal models (LMMs)

Generalist LLMs such as GPT-4 have demonstrated astonishing capabilities in various health applications, but they still have significant growth areas. In multimodal generative AI, the potential gap in health competency may be even larger, as there is scarce availability of multimodal, longitudinal health data in the public web for pretraining.

Contrastive learning

A standard approach to multimodal learning is contrastive learning. Contrastive learning has a long history in NLP and computer vision, initially focusing on unimodal scenarios (e.g., by creating semantic-equivalent variants of an image and training the encoder to map them closer to each other). It can be extended to the multimodal regime by pushing corresponding instances across modalities (e.g., image-text pairs) closer and non-corresponding ones farther apart, akin to machine translation.

To sustain and accelerate progress in health generative AI, it is thus important to invest in comprehensive benchmark creation and evaluation that represent diverse populations and real-world scenarios.

For precision health, a major bottleneck lies in the scarcity of biomedical data in common resources for multimodal pretraining. One way to address this deficiency is by extracting cross-modal data from publicly available resources. By extracting biomedical figures and their corresponding captions and citations from PubMed-Central articles, the BiomedCLIP project has assembled one of the largest datasets for biomedical vision-language pretraining, with 15 million image-text pairs across diverse categories and 46 million fine-grained pairs after splitting composite figures.

Standard contrastive learning treats all modalities equally. In practice, text captures a large swath of digitized knowledge, whereas data for other modalities is much scarcer by comparison. Multimodal input is tokenized and embedded in the natural-language instruction for output generation by a large language model. Subsequent biomedical large multimodal models (such as MedPaLM-M) all follow the same general recipe to align image and text, but LLaVA-Med stands out by using GPT-4 to generate multimodal instruction-following data. Similar approaches can also be applied to other modalities such as single-cell data and protein sequences.

Ultimately, routinely collected real-world clinical data represents the biggest growth opportunity for multimodal generative AI. For example, a cancer patient may have hundreds of clinical notes with their corresponding imaging, multi-omics, and other medical tests, across the disease trajectory from diagnosis to treatment to outcome. Such naturally occurring multimodal, longitudinal data can be leveraged to bridge the health competency gap in LLMs, following the general recipe of LLaVA-Med.

Ongoing research in digital pathology exploration has demonstrated promise. Researchers have collaborated to train real-world pathology foundation models using over one billion images from hundreds of thousands of slides along with clinical reports, with initial promising results in pathomics and progression modelling. Meanwhile, the BiomedJourney project extended the LLaVA-Med approach to image generation, by using GPT-4 to generate instruction-following data from multimodal patient journeys. This enables BiomedJourney to help answer what-if questions for in silico medical imaging.

By encapsulating multimodal and longitudinal dependencies from population-level real-world data, LMMs can potentially unlock a slew of high-value applications, from cross-modal retrieval and generation, to multimodal conversational copilots (enabling stakeholders to "talk to" multimodal data), to the ultimate dream of precision health: learning from multimodal real-world observational data to predict longitudinal treatment outcome and adverse events.

The AI market in healthcare is estimated to grow from a $5 billion industry in 2020 to $45 billion in 2026.

NEOPLASTIC DISEASES

Chapter 3. Breast cancer

- Use of AI to improve radiologists' interpretation of mammograms for diagnosing breast cancer

In a retrospective study an AI algorithm was developed and validated with 170,230 mammography examinations collected from five institutions in South Korea, the USA, and the UK, including 36,468 which were cancer-positive confirmed by biopsy,

59,544 which were benign confirmed by biopsy (8,827 mammograms) or follow-up imaging (50,717 mammograms), and 74,218 which were normal. The performance of AI and that of radiologists was evaluated in terms of the area under the receiver operating characteristic curve (AUROC) and recall-based sensitivity and specificity.

AI performed better than the radiologists, particularly with cancers demonstrating a mass, distortion or asymmetry. AI was also better at detecting early cancers and lymph-node negative cancers. The performance of radiologists improved when they used AI as a supportive diagnostic tool.[27]

- A deep learning algorithm to improve pathologist accuracy and efficiency

The investigators conducted a multi-reader, multi-case study utilizing a deep learning algorithm for the detection of breast cancer metastasis in lymph nodes. Six pathologists reviewed 70 digitized slides from lymph node sections. Algorithm-assisted pathologists had increased accuracy than pathologists without algorithm assistance, especially for the detection of micrometastases. Review time was shorter when pathologists were assisted by the algorithm.[38]

- Deep learning algorithms for analysis of whole-slide pathology images can potentially improve diagnostic accuracy and efficiency.

Investigators developed a series of deep learning algorithms for reading hematoxylin and eosin-stained tissue sections of lymph nodes of women with breast cancer and compared the results with those of pathologists. The presence of specific metastatic foci and the absence vs presence of lymph node metastasis in a slide was measured using receiver operating characteristic curve analysis. For the whole-slide image classification task, the best algorithm performed significantly better than the pathologists. Whether this approach has clinical utility will require evaluation in a clinical setting.[39]

- The importance of external validation of an ensemble model for automated mammography interpretation by artificial intelligence[49]

The investigators aimed to externally validate an ensemble deep-learning model using data from a high-volume, distributed screening program of an academic health system with a diverse patient population.In this diagnostic study, an ensemble learning method, which reweights outputs of the 11 highest-performing individual AI models from the Digital Mammography Dialogue on Reverse Engineering Assessment and Methods (DREAM) Mammography Challenge, was used to predict the cancer status of an individual using a standard set of screening mammography images. Performance of the challenge ensemble method (CEM) and the CEM combined with radiologist assessment (CEM+R) were compared with regard to diagnosed ductal carcinoma in situ and invasive cancers within a year of the screening examination using performance metrics, such as sensitivity, specificity, and area under the receiver operating characteristic curve (AUROC). The study evaluated 37,317 examinations from 26,817 women. Individual model AUROC estimates ranged from 0.77 to 0.83. The CEM model achieved an AUROC of 0.85 in the UCLA cohort, which was lower than the performance achieved in the Kaiser Permanente Washington (AUROC, 0.90) and Karolinska Institute (AUROC, 0.92) cohorts. The CEM+R model achieved a sensitivity and specificity, which was similar to that of the radiologists' performance. The investigators concluded that the high performance of an ensemble deep-learning model for automated screening mammography interpretation did not generalize to a more diverse screening cohort, suggesting that the model experienced underspecification. This study suggests the need for model transparency and fine-tuning of AI models for specific target populations prior to their clinical adoption.

Chapter 4. Lung cancer and lung nodules detected on chest x-rays

Several studies have found AI to be of use in the evaluation of pulmonary nodules detected on chest x-rays.[21 – 24]

- AI Improves nodule detection on chest radiographs in a health screening population: a randomized controlled trial

For example, in a study by Yoo et al.[23] a total of 5,485 participants were included, with a median follow-up duration of 6.5 years. This diagnostic study assessed the performance of a deep learning–based AI algorithm for the detection of pulmonary nodules and lung cancer on chest radiographs. In this study, the sensitivity and specificity of an artificial intelligence algorithm for nodule detection were 86% and 85%, respectively. When the same artificial intelligence algorithm was applied for cancer detection, the sensitivity was 94%, specificity 83%, for the detection of malignant pulmonary nodules. The AI algorithm performed better than the National Lung Cancer Screening Trial (NLST) radiologists for the detection of all noncalcified nodules and malignant pulmonary nodules on digital radiographs. This AI algorithm may help to detect lung cancer by detecting additional malignant pulmonary nodules.

Chapter 5. Colo-rectal cancer (CRC)

Several studies have found AI-assisted colonoscopy to improve the colonic adenoma detection rate. Adenomas can subsequently transform to malignant colon cancers[30,65]

- An automatic polyp detection system during colonoscopy resulted in a significant increase in the number of diminutive adenomas detected, as well as an increase in the rate of hyperplastic polyps.[30]

The effect of colonoscopy on colorectal cancer mortality is limited by a miss rate, leading to decreased adenoma detection rates. Adenomas can subsequently become malignant. The investigators compared the colonoscopy-detection rate of adenomas with versus without an automatic polyp detection system. The artificial intelligence system significantly increased the adenoma detection rate and the mean number of adenomas per patient. In addition, the number of hyperplastic polyps was also significantly increased using AI-assisted colonoscopy. The cost-benefit ratio of such effects has to be determined further.

Chapter 6. Urologic diseases including prostate cancer

Two literature reviews have been published on the use of AI in urologic diseases.[31,32]

- AI will change the landscape of urological cancer management

One group of investigators searched the PubMed-MEDLINE databases for articles in English on machine learning (ML) and deep learning (DL) models related to general surgery and prostate, bladder, and kidney cancer. The search terms were a combination of keywords, including both "urology" and "artificial intelligence" with one of the following: "machine learning," "deep learning," "neural network," "renal cell carcinoma," "kidney cancer," "urothelial carcinoma," "bladder cancer," "prostate cancer," and "robotic surgery."

Studies on prostate cancer were related to the prediction of grade, improved diagnosis, and prediction of outcomes and of recurrence. Studies on bladder cancer mainly used radiomics to identify aggressive tumors and predict treatment outcomes, recurrence and survival rates. Most studies on the application of ML and DL in kidney cancer were focused on the differentiation of benign and malignant tumors as well as prediction of their grade and subtype. Most studies suggested that methods using AI may be better than or similar to existing traditional methods.

The authors concluded that, despite technological, legal, and ethical concerns, AI will change the landscape of urological cancer management.[31]

- The continuous incorporation of clinical data, further ML and DL algorithm retraining, and generalizability of models will augment prediction accuracy and enhance individualized medicine.[32]

The authors conducted a search of original articles using the PubMed MEDLINE database to identify recent English literature relevant to machine learning (ML) and deep learning (DL) applications in the fields of urolithiasis, renal cell carcinoma (RCC), bladder cancer, and prostate cancer.

They found that the most common ML and DL application in urolithiasis is in the prediction of endourologic surgical outcomes. The main area of research involving ML and DL in RCC concerned the differentiation between benign and malignant small renal masses, Fuhrman nuclear grade prediction, and gene expression-based molecular signatures. For bladder cancer they found that studies employed radiomics and texture feature analysis for the distinction between low- and high-grade tumors, addressed accurate image-based cytology, and used algorithms to predict treatment response, tumor recurrence, and patient survival. For prostate cancer they found that studies aimed at developing algorithms for Gleason score prediction, MRI computer-aided diagnosis, and surgical outcomes and biochemical recurrence prediction. Studies consistently found the superiority of these methods over traditional statistical methods.

Chapter 7. Skin cancer

- Artificial intelligence and machine learning algorithms for early detection of skin cancer in community and primary care settings: a systematic review[1]

The investigators reviewed studies on artificial intelligence and machine learning algorithms that aimed to facilitate the early diagnosis of skin cancers in primary and community care settings. The primary outcomes showed a mean diagnostic accuracy for melanoma (89·5%), squamous cell carcinoma (85·3%), and basal cell carcinoma (87·6%).

- The authors classified skin lesions using a single convolutional neural network (CNN) trained on129,450 clinical images and compared its performance with that of 21 board-certified dermatologists on biopsy-proven clinical images of
  1. Keratinocyte carcinomas versus benign seborrheic keratoses
  2. Malignant melanomas versus benign nevi.

  The CNN's performance was on par with that of the dermatologists across both tasks, demonstrating that artificial intelligence is capable of classifying skin cancer with a level of competence comparable to that of dermatologists. It is projected that 6.3 billion smartphone subscriptions will exist by the year 2021 and could therefore potentially provide low-cost universal access to vital dermatologic diagnostic care.[43] (Editorial note: the number of smart phones globally in 2024 is anticipated to be 7 million. The global human population in 2024 is 8.2 million).

Chapter 8. Gastric cancer

- Predicting peritoneal recurrence and disease-free survival from CT images in gastric cancer with multitask deep learning: a retrospective study[19]

The authors aimed to develop predictive models for peritoneal recurrence of gastric cancer and the prognosis of gastric cancer. They performed a retrospective multi-institution study of 2,320 patients to develop a multitask deep learning model for the simultaneous prediction of peritoneal recurrence and disease-free survival using preoperative CT images. They assessed whether the model could improve the ability of clinicians to predict peritoneal recurrence. In multivariable analysis the model predicted peritoneal recurrence and disease-free survival independently of clinicopathological variables ($p<0{\cdot}0001$ for all). For patients with a predicted high risk of peritoneal recurrence and low survival, adjuvant chemotherapy was associated with improved disease-free survival in both stage II disease and stage III disease. Chemotherapy was found to have no impact on disease-free survival for patients with a predicted low risk of peritoneal recurrence and high survival. For the remaining patients, the benefit of chemotherapy depended on stage: only those with stage III disease derived benefit from chemotherapy.

Prospective studies are required to test the clinical utility of this model in guiding personalised treatment in combination with clinicopathological criteria.

Chapter 9. Brain cancer

- Deep learning for segmentation of brain tumors: impact of cross-institutional training and testing[50]

The investigators assessed the effect of cross-institutional training on the performance of convolutional neural networks (CNNs), which are commonly used for segmentation of brain tumors on imaging. They selected 44 cases of glioblastoma multiforme from two institutions in The Cancer Imaging Archive dataset. The images were manually annotated by outlining each tumor component to form ground truth. To automatically segment the tumors in each patient, they trained three CNNs: (a) one using data for patients from the same institution as the test data, (b) one using data for the patients from the other institution and (c) one using data for the patients from both of the institutions. Performance of the model significantly decreased ($P < 0.0001$) when it was trained on data from a different institution as compared to training with data from the same institution. This trend persisted for segmentation of the entire tumor as well as its individual components. There is a very strong effect of selecting data for training on performance of CNNs in a multi-institutional setting.

Determination of the reasons behind this effect requires additional comprehensive investigation.

Chapter 10. Cancer of unknown primary site

- AI-based pathology slides can predict the origins for cancers of unknown primary site[3]

Cancer of unknown primary origin is an enigmatic group of diagnoses in which the primary anatomical site of tumour origin cannot be determined. Investigators developed a deep learning-based algorithm called Tumour Origin Assessment via Deep Learning (TOAD), that was able to provide a differential diagnosis for the origin of the primary tumour using routinely acquired histology slides. They used whole-slide images of tumours with known primary origins to train a model that simultaneously identified the tumour as primary or metastatic and predicted its site of origin. The model achieved a top-1 accuracy of 0.83 and a top-3 accuracy of 0.96.

NON-NEOPLASTIC DISEASES

Chapter 11. Cerebrovascular diseases

- Deep learning-assisted diagnosis of cerebral aneurysms using the HeadXNet model[52]

The investigators developed and applied a neural network segmentation model (the HeadXNet model) capable of generating precise voxel-by-voxel predictions of intracranial aneurysms on computed tomographic angiography (CTA) imaging of the head in order to augment the diagnostic performance of clinicians for intracranial aneurysms. A convolutional neural network architecture was developed using a training set of 611 head CTA examinations to generate aneurysm segmentations. Head and neck examinations performed between January 3, 2003 and May 31, 2017 at a single academic medical center were used to train, validate, and test the model. Examinations positive for aneurysm had at least 1 clinically significant, nonruptured intracranial aneurysm. The data set contained 818 examinations from 662 patients with 328 CTA examinations containing at least 1 intracranial aneurysm and 490 examinations without intracranial aneurysms. The radiology experience of the clinicians reading the test set ranged from 2 to 12 years. Augmenting clinicians with artificial intelligence-produced segmentation predictions resulted in clinicians achieving statistically significant improvements in sensitivity, accuracy, and interrater agreement when compared with no augmentation. The clinicians' mean sensitivity increased by 0.059, mean accuracy increased by 0.038, and mean interrater agreement increased by 0.060, from 0.799 to 0.859. The investigators concluded thar their deep learning model successfully detected clinically significant intracranial aneurysms on CTA. This suggested that integration of an artificial intelligence-assisted diagnostic model may augment clinician diagnosis of intracranial aneurisms with dependable and accurate predictions and thereby optimize patient care.

- The use of AI to detect emergent large vessel occlusion (ELVO) improved clinically meaningful stroke workflow metrics, resulting in faster treatment times for mechanical thrombectomy.[9]

Six hundred and eighty consecutive strokes were evaluated by AI. 104 patients were diagnosed with emergent large vessel occlusion (ELVO). Forty-five patients with ELVO were identified by AI and 59 by normal standard of care. Sixty-nine mechanical thrombectomies were performed. The median time from computed tomography angiography (CTA) to team notification was shorter for AI ELVOs (7 vs 26 min; $p<0.001$). Door to arterial puncture was faster for transfer patients with ELVO detected by AI versus usual care transfer patients (141 vs 185 min; $p=0.027$). AI yielded a time savings of 22 min for team notification and a 23 min reduction in door to arterial puncture for transfer patients. AI automated alerts can be incorporated into a comprehensive stroke center hub and spoke system of care.

- Development and validation of a set of deep learning algorithms for the automated detection of strokes or head trauma on non-contrast CT scans[40]

Key findings on the CT scans were intracranial hemorrhage and its types (intraparenchymal, intraventricular, subdural, extradural, and subarachnoid); calvarial fractures; midline shift; and mass effect. The retrospective dataset contained

313,318 head CT scans together with their clinical reports from 20 centres in India. A randomly selected part of this dataset (Qure25k dataset) was used for validation and the rest was used to develop algorithms. An additional validation dataset (CQ500 dataset) was collected in two batches from centres that were different from those used for the development and Qure25k datasets. Areas under the receiver operating characteristic curves (AUROCs) were used to assess the algorithms. The Qure25k dataset contained 21,095 scans and the CQ500 dataset consisted of 214 scans in the first batch and 277 scans in the second batch. On the Qure25k dataset, the algorithms achieved an AUROC of 0·92 for detecting intracranial hemorrhage, 0·90 for intraparenchymal hemorrhage, 0·96 for intraventricular hemorrhage, 0·92 for subdural hemorrhage, 0·93 for extradural hemorrhage, and 0·90 for subarachnoid hemorrhage. AUROCs on the Qure25k dataset were 0·92 for calvaria fractures, 0·93 for midline shift, and 0·86 for mass effect. The investigators concluded that deep learning algorithms accurately identify head CT scan abnormalities requiring urgent attention, opening up the possibility of using these algorithms to automate the triage process.

- Evaluation of a DL model for the automatic detection of intracranial hemorrhage and its subtypes on non-contrast CT head studies and comparison of the effects of various preprocessing and model design implementations.[41]

The DL algorithm was trained and externally validated on open-source, multi-centre retrospective data containing radiologist-annotated non-contrast CT head studies. The training dataset was sourced from four research institutions across Canada, the USA and Brazil. The test dataset was sourced from a research centre in India. A convolutional neural network (CNN) was used, with its performance compared against similar models with additional implementations: (1) a recurrent neural network (RNN) attached to the CNN, (2) preprocessed CT image-windowed inputs and (3) preprocessed CT image-concatenated (not linked) inputs. The area under the receiver operating characteristic curve (AUCROC) and microaveraged precision (mAP) score were used to evaluate and compare model performances. The training and test datasets contained 21,744 and 491 non-contrast CT head studies, respectively, with 8,882 (40.8%) and 205 (41.8%) positive for intracranial hemorrhage. Implementation of preprocessing techniques and the CNN-RNN framework increased mAP from 0.77 to 0.93 and increased AUCROC from 0.854 to

0.966 (p-value = 3.91×10^{-12}). The investigators concluded that the deep learning model accurately detected intracranial hemorrhage and improved in performance following specific implementation techniques, demonstrating clinical potential as a decision support tool and an automated system to improve radiologist workflow efficiency.

Chapter 11. Cardiovascular diseases

- AI reading of EKGs facilitates treatment time in people with STEMI[12]

Electrocardiograms (EKGs in the USA or ECGs in some other countries) give a visible read-out of the conduction of electrical currents in the heart which then stimulate the atria and ventricles to contract, thus enabling circulation of the blood. There are several abnormalities of the EKG in people who are suffering an acute myocardial infarction (AMI).

The appearance of a normal EKG is shown in Figure 1.

Figure 1. Schematic diagram of normal sinus rhythm for a human heart as seen on an EKG

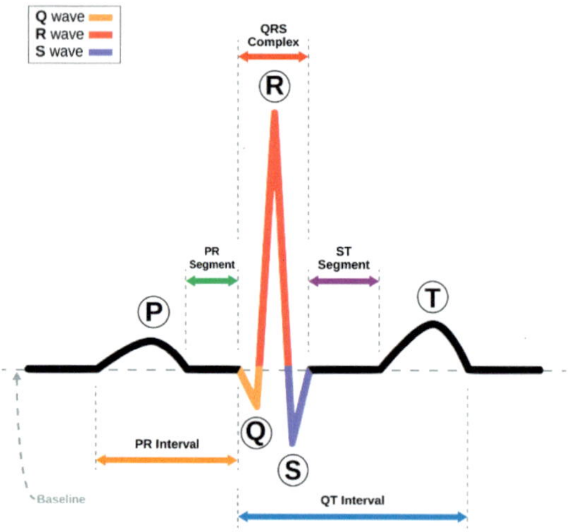

This image is by Created by Agateller (Anthony Atkielski), converted to svg by atom. - SinusRhythmLabels.png, Public Domain, https://commons.wikimedia.org/w/index.php?curid=1560893; en.wikipedia.org/wiki/Electrocardiography#/media/File:SinusRhythmLabels.svg. The copyright holder of this image has released it into the public domain. No changes were made to this image

One abnormality of the EKG that occurs in some people experiencing an AMI is elevation of the ST segment of the EKG.

Figure 2. Illustration of ST segment elevation

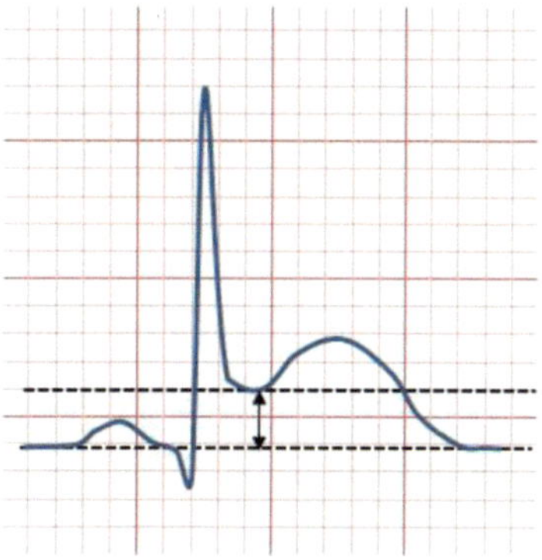

Such cases are known as ST elevation in myocardial infarction (STEMI). A study published in 2024 showed that AI-assisted EKGs could detect ST segment elevation in AMI patients more quickly than non-AI-assisted EKGs and that this led to a decreased door-to-balloon time for patients presenting to the emergency department and decreased the EKG-to-balloon time for patients in the emergency room and inpatients. However, the study did not indicate whether this impacted on clinical treatment and patient outcome.

(Editorial note: an inflatable ballon inserted into the blocked coronary artery is one method of restoring blood flow in the blocked artery; metal stents are an alternative to balloons for this purpose).

- Convolutional neural networks (CNNs) have been developed to detect asymptomatic left ventricular dysfunction, silent atrial fibrillation, hypertrophic cardiomyopathy and an individual's age, sex and race on the basis of the EKG alone[2].

- Coronary artery calcium (CAC) as assessed by computed tomography (CT) is a marker of subclinical coronary atherosclerosis. Investigators developed an AI-enabled EKG framework that only predicted a CAC score ≥400 [4].

- A different group of investigators presented two deep learning models that automated coronary artery calcium (CAC) scoring and which demonstrated advantages in automated scoring for both dedicated gated coronary artery CT examinations and routine non-gated chest CTs performed for other reasons. They first trained a gated coronary artery CT model for CAC scoring that showed near perfect agreement with current conventional manual scoring on a retrospective dataset of 79 patients. Then, using CAC scores from paired gated coronary artery CT examinations as a reference standard, they trained a deep learning model on their internal data and a cohort from the Multi-Ethnic Study of Atherosclerosis study to perform CAC scoring on routine non-gated chest CT exams with validation on external datasets obtained from four geographically disparate health systems. When identifying patients with any CAC score (i.e., CAC score≥ 1), sensitivity and positive predictive value were high across all datasets. For CAC scores ≥ 100 on routine non-gated chest CTs, which is the most recent recommended threshold to initiate statin therapy, their model showed sensitivities of 71-94% and positive predictive values in the range of 88-100% across all the sites. Adoption of this model could allow more patients to be screened with CAC scoring, potentially allowing earlier preventive interventions.[25]

- Investigators developed three convolutional neural networks (CNNs) to evaluate their performance in interpreting left ventricular (LV) function obtained from short-axis cine magnetic resonance images (MRIs).

The LV function parameters derived from one CNN (CNN3) showed a high correlation ($r^2 \geq 0.98$) and agreement with those obtained by experts. A deep learning-based method trained on a data set with high variability can achieve fully automated and accurate cine MRI analysis on multivendor, multicenter cine MRI data.[8]

- An AI algorithm is a viable tool for detecting even mild hyperkalemia from a two-lead EKG.[42]

Hyperkalemia is commonly seen in congestive heart failure, chronic kidney disease, diabetes mellitus and with the medications used to treat these conditions. It is associated with significant mortality and arrhythmic risk. Electrocardiogram (EKG) changes in hyperkalemia are clearly visible only in severe cases. Because it is frequently asymptomatic, detecting hyperkalemia is challenging, and requires access to blood. Data from patients seen between 1994 and 2017 with a serum potassium acquired within 12 hours of an EKG were included in this study. Study data included 709,000 patients, 2.1 million EKGs and 4.0 million serum potassium values. Patients were split randomly into training (2/3) and testing (1/3) groups. A threshold of 5.0 mmol/L was used for hyperkalemia and false positives were eliminated by selecting for repeated positive tests, resulting in 20,196 positive and 2.0 million negative samples. An artificial intelligence (AI) algorithm utilizing a deep neural network was trained to detect hyperkalemia using only EKG leads I and II. Performance was evaluated on the testing group. An additional, prospective, independent testing dataset was also obtained in 10 patients undergoing hemodialysis.

In the first testing group of 698,939 EKGs from 224,690 patients, the AUC was 0.87 (sensitivity 85%, specificity 72%). In the dialysis group the sensitivity by duration was 94% and specificity was 74%. The investigators concluded that their AI algorithm was a viable tool for detecting even mild hyperkalemia from a two-lead EKG. In combination with a smartphone EKG, this may enable a new means for rapid, non-invasive monitoring and screening for hyperkalemia at home and in the clinic.

- Retinal imaging biomarkers for cardiovascular disease[37]

The accessibility of the retina with the use of non-invasive and relatively low-cost ophthalmic imaging techniques and analytics provides a unique opportunity to improve the detection, diagnosis and monitoring of systemic diseases. The National Heart, Lung, and Blood Institute of the National Institutes of Health USA examined this concept and developed a Roadmap from its findings. This Roadmap describes new research opportunities to evaluate the relationships between the eye (in particular, retinal biomarkers) and the risk of cardiovascular diseases, including coronary artery disease, heart failure, stroke, hypertension and cerebrovascular dementia. Identified gaps included the need to simplify and standardize the capture of high-quality images of the eye by non-ophthalmic health workers and to conduct longitudinal studies using multidisciplinary networks of diverse at-risk populations with improved implementation. Future research on retinal microvascular disease and retinal biomarkers might provide insights into the temporal development of microvascular disease across other systemic vascular beds.

- Prediction of cardiovascular risk factors from retinal fundus photographs using deep learning[64]

Investigators showed that deep learning can extract new knowledge from retinal fundus images. Using deep-learning models trained on data from 284,335 patients and validated on two independent datasets of 12,026 and 999 patients, they predicted cardiovascular risk factors not previously thought to be present or quantifiable in retinal images, such as age (mean absolute error within 3.26 years), gender (area under the receiver operating characteristic curve (AUC) = 0.97), smoking status (AUC = 0.71), systolic blood pressure (mean absolute error within 11.23 mmHg) and major adverse cardiac events (AUC = 0.70). They also showed that the trained deep-learning models used anatomical features, such as the optic disc or blood vessels, to generate each prediction.

Chapter 29. Neurologic diseases

- Investigators found that a deep learning model of head CT and clinical information can be used to predict 6-month outcomes after severe traumatic brain injury.[10]

- An AI application that is targeted for use by non-radiologist clinicians for detecting large-vessel occlusions in the central nervous system has resulted in a significant reduction in time to intervention and improved patient outcomes.[20]

- Neuroimaging modality fusion in Alzheimer's classification using convolutional neural networks[26]

Automated methods for Alzheimer's disease (AD) classification have the potential for great clinical benefits and may provide insight for combating the disease. Machine learning, and more specifically deep neural networks, have been shown to have great efficacy in this domain. These algorithms often use neurological imaging data such as those from MRI and FDG PET scans, but a comprehensive and balanced comparison of the MRI and amyloid PET modalities has not been performed. In order to accurately determine the relative strength of each imaging variant, these investigators performed a comparison study in the context of Alzheimer's dementia classification using the Alzheimer's Disease Neuroimaging Initiative (ADNI) dataset with identical neural network architectures. Furthermore, this work analyzed the benefits of using both modalities in a fusion setting and discussed how these data types may be leveraged in future AD studies using deep learning.

Chapter 14. Pulmonary diseases

- The use of AI in the detection of pneumothorax[10]

Analysis of one study included radiographs from 985 patients including 307 patients with a nontension pneumothorax, 128 patients with tension pneumothorax, and 550 patients without pneumothorax. The AI model detected any pneumothorax with an AUC of 0.979, sensitivity of 94.3%, and specificity of 92.0% and tension pneumothorax with an AUC of 0.987, sensitivity of 94.5%, and specificity of 95.3%. These findings suggest that the assessed AI model accurately detected pneumothorax and tension pneumothorax in this chest radiograph data set. The model's use in the clinical workflow could lead to earlier identification and improved care for patients with pneumothorax.[10]

- Artificial intelligence augmentation of radiologists' performance in distinguishing COVID-19 from pneumonia of other origin on chest CT scans[47]

The investigators sought to establish and evaluate an artificial intelligence system for differentiating COVID-19 and other pneumonia on chest CT scanning and assessing radiologist performance without and with AI assistance. A total of 521 patients with positive reverse transcription polymerase chain reaction results for COVID-19 and abnormal chest CT findings were retrospectively identified from 10 hospitals from January 2020 to April 2020. A total of 665 patients with non-COVID-19 pneumonia and definite evidence of pneumonia at chest CT were retrospectively selected from three hospitals between 2017 and 2019. To classify COVID-19 versus other pneumonia for each patient, abnormal CT slices were inputted into the EfficientNet B4 deep neural network architecture after lung segmentation, followed by a two-layer fully connected neural network to pool slices together. The final cohort of 1,186 patients (132,583 CT slices) was divided into training, validation, and test sets in a 7:2:1 and equal ratio. Independent testing was performed by evaluating the model's performance in separate hospitals. Studies were blindly reviewed by six radiologists without and then with AI assistance. The final model achieved a test accuracy of 96%, a sensitivity of 95%, and a specificity of 96% with area under the receiver operating characteristic curve of 0.95 and area under the precision-recall curve of 0.90. On independent testing, this model achieved an accuracy of 87%, a sensitivity of 89%, and a specificity of 86% with area under the receiver operating characteristic curve of 0.90 and area under the precision-recall curve of 0.87. Assisted by the AI model, the radiologists achieved a higher average test accuracy, sensitivity, and specificity.

- A case-study in the detection of pulmonary embolism[56]

The investigators developed and compared different multimodal fusion model architectures that were capable of utilizing both pixel data from volumetric computed tomography pulmonary angiography scans and clinical patient data from the electronic medical record to automatically classify cases of pulmonary embolism. The best performing multimodality model ws a late fusion model that achieved an AUROC of 0.947 on the entire test set, outperforming imaging-only and EMR-only single modality models.

- Machine learning and deep neural network applications in the thorax: pulmonary embolism, chronic thromboembolic pulmonary hypertension, aorta, and chronic obstructive pulmonary disease[57]

The radiologic community is rapidly integrating a revolution that has not fully entered daily practice. It necessitates a close collaboration between computer scientists and radiologists to move from concepts to practical applications. The investigators reviewed the current literature on machine learning and deep neural network applications in the field of pulmonary embolism, chronic thromboembolic pulmonary hypertension, aorta, and chronic obstructive pulmonary disease.

- Identifying medical diagnoses and treatable diseases by image-based deep learning.[62]

Kermany et al developed an artificial intelligence system using transfer learning techniques. It accurately distinguished bacterial and viral pneumonia on chest X-rays.

- Artificial intelligence (AI)-assisted diagnosis imparted high accuracy to chest radiography (CXR) interpretation.[45]

The investigators randomly allocated eligible patients who visited an outpatient clinic to an intervention (with AI-assisted interpretation) or control (without AI-assisted interpretation) groups. Lung lesions on CXR were recorded by seven non-radiologists with or without AI assistance. The reference standard for lung lesions was established by three radiologists. The primary and secondary endpoints were the physicians' diagnostic accuracy and clinical decision, respectively. 162 and 161 patients were assigned to the intervention and control groups, respectively. The area under the receiver operating characteristic curve (AUROC) was significantly larger in the intervention group than in the control group for the CXR level and lung lesion level. The intervention group had higher sensitivity in terms of both CXR and lung lesion level and a lower false referral rate for the lung lesion level. The investigators concluded that AI-assisted CXR interpretation improved the diagnostic performance of non-radiologist physicians in detecting abnormal lung findings.[4]

- Artificial intelligence algorithm detecting lung infection in supine chest radiographs of critically ill patients[46]

In a retrospective study the investigators evaluated a prototype artificial intelligence algorithm to classify basal lung opacities according to underlying pathologies. The deep neural network was trained on two publicly available datasets including 297,541 images of 86,876 patients. One hundred sixty-six patients received both supine chest radiograph and CT scans within 90 minutes without any intervention in between. The algorithm accuracy was referenced to board-certified radiologists who evaluated supine chest radiographs according to reading scores for pneumonia and effusion (0 = absent, 1 = possible, and 2 = highly suspected). Performances of radiologists and the artificial intelligence algorithm were quantified by receiver-operating characteristic curve analysis (AUROC). With regard to pneumonia detection, radiologists achieved a maximum diagnostic accuracy of up to 0.87 when considering only the supine chest radiograph. With regard to the detection of pleural effusions, there was no significant performance difference between the radiologists' performance and that of the artificial intelligence algorithm. The investigators concluded that artificial intelligence is a promising clinical decision support tool for supine chest radiograph examinations.

- CheXaid: a deep learning assistance for physician diagnosis of tuberculosis using chest x-rays in patients with HIV[54]

Tuberculosis (TB) is the leading cause of preventable death in HIV-positive patients, and yet often remains undiagnosed and untreated. Chest x-ray is often used to assist in diagnosis, yet this presents additional challenges due to atypical radiographic presentation and radiologist shortages in regions where co-infection is most common. The investigators developed a deep learning algorithm to diagnose TB using clinical information and chest x-ray images from 677 HIV-positive patients with suspected TB from two hospitals in South Africa. They then sought to determine whether the algorithm could assist clinicians in the diagnosis of TB in HIV-positive patients as a web-based diagnostic assistant. Use of the algorithm resulted in a modest but statistically significant improvement in clinician accuracy, increasing the mean clinician accuracy from 0.60 without assistance to 0.65 with assistance.

However, the accuracy of assisted clinicians was significantly lower than that of the stand-alone algorithm, which had an accuracy of 0.79 on the same unseen test cases. These results suggested that deep learning assistance may improve clinician accuracy in the diagnosis of TB using chest x-rays, which would be valuable in settings with a high burden of HIV/TB co-infection. Moreover, the high accuracy of the stand-alone algorithm suggests a potential value particularly in settings with a scarcity of radiological expertise.

Chapter 15. Infectious diseases

- Advances in artificial intelligence for infectious-disease surveillance

The investigators reviewed the effects of new and long-standing AI solutions for infectious-disease surveillance. AI applications have been shown to be successful for a diverse set of functions, including early-warning systems, hotspot detection, epidemiologic tracking and forecasting, and resource allocation.

- Autonomous AI systems that use a robotic nonmydriatic fundus camera with a built-in AI algorithm to provide feedback to the operator to acquire high-quality fundus photographs for determining the presence or absence of referable diabetic eye disease (DED), with immediate results after image acquisition at the point of care, have been developed[4].

Chapter 16. Ophthalmology

- An AI system for the diagnosis of diabetic retinopathy (DR) and diabetic macular edema (DME)[4]

In a pivotal trial an autonomous AI system demonstrated 87% sensitivity and 90% specificity in detecting DR and/or DME in adults with diabetes mellitus. The autonomous AI system guided the operator to acquire two color fundus images determined to be of adequate quality using an image quality algorithm, with one cantered on the fovea and the other on the optic nerve. This system developed by Luminetics Digital Diagnostics was the first autonomous system approved by the USA Food and Drug Administration.

- Use of adjudication to quantify errors in diabetic retinopathy (DR) grading based on individual graders and majority decision, and to train an improved automated algorithm for DR grading[33].

This retrospective study compared the diagnosis of diabetic retinopathy graded by a previously developed AI algorithm with that by ophthalmologists and retinal experts. The investigators found that the most common discrepancies were missing microaneurysms, artifacts, and misclassified hemorrhages. For moderate or worse DR, the majority decision of ophthalmologists had a sensitivity of 0.838 and specificity of 0.981. The algorithm had a sensitivity of 0.971, and a specificity of 0.923. The authors concluded that by using a small number of adjudicated consensus grades as a tuning dataset and higher-resolution images as input, the algorithm improved in AUC from 0.934 to 0.986 for moderate or worse DR. The resulting algorithm's performance was on par with that of individual U.S.A. Board-certified ophthalmologists and retinal specialists.

- Deep learning algorithms can improve the accuracy of, and confidence in, the diagnosis of DR diagnosis in an assisted read setting[35]

In this study the investigators included 1,796 retinal fundus images from 1,612 patients with diabetes mellitus. Ten ophthalmologists read images for DR severity based on the International Clinical Diabetic Retinopathy disease severity scale in each of 3 conditions: unassisted, grades only, or grades plus heatmap. Grades-only assistance comprised a histogram of DR predictions (grades) from a trained deep-learning model. For grades plus heatmap, we additionally showed explanatory heatmaps.

The ophthalmologists graded DR more accurately with model assistance than without for the grades-only condition. Grades plus heatmaps improved accuracy for patients with DR, but reduced accuracy for patients without DR.

- The application of deep learning to create an algorithm for automated detection of diabetic retinopathy in retinal fundus photographs.[36]

A convolutional neural network was trained using a retrospective data set of 128,175 retinal images, which were graded 3 to 7 times for diabetic retinopathy, diabetic macular edema, and image gradability by a panel of 54 US licensed ophthalmologists and ophthalmology senior residents. The algorithm was evaluated from the development data set, one selected for high specificity and another for high sensitivity. The algorithm based on deep machine learning had high sensitivity and specificity for detecting referable diabetic retinopathy. Further research is necessary to determine the feasibility of applying this algorithm in the clinical setting and to determine whether use of the algorithm could lead to improved care and outcomes compared with current ophthalmologic assessment.[36]

- A deep learning-based segmentation tool provided clinically useful measures of retinal disease that would otherwise would have been able to obtain.[44]

Quantitative volumetric measures of retinal disease using optical coherence tomography (OCT) scans are infeasible due to the time required for manual grading. The authors evaluated a deep learning model for whole-volume segmentation of 4 clinically important pathological features and assess clinical applicability.This diagnostic study used OCT data from 173 patients with a total of 15,558 B-scans, treated at Moorfields Eye Hospital in London. The data set included 2 macular conditions: wet age-related macular degeneration (107 scans) and diabetic macular edema (66 scans), covering the full range of severity. Two expert graders performed pixel-level segmentations of intraretinal fluid, subretinal fluid, subretinal hyperreflective material, and pigment epithelial detachment, including all B-scans in each OCT volume, taking as long as 50 hours per scan. Among the 173 patients included in the analysis qualitative assessment found that automated whole-volume segmentation ranked better than, or comparable to, at least 1 expert grader in 127 scans. The model was rated neutrally or positively in 86% to 92% of diabetic macular edema scans and 53% to 87% of age-related macular degeneration scans. The authors concluded that the deep learning-based segmentation tool provided clinically useful measures of retinal disease that would otherwise have not have been feasible to obtain. Qualitative evaluation was additionally important to reveal clinical applicability for both care management and research.

- Identifying medical diagnoses and treatable diseases by image-based deep learning[62]

Kermany et al developed an artificial intelligence system using transfer learning techniques. It effectively classified images for macular degeneration and diabetic retinopathy.

Chapter 17. Obstetrics

- AI estimation of gestational age from blind ultrasound sweeps in low-resource settings[48]

Ultrasound is indispensable to gestational age estimation and thus to quality obstetrical care, yet high equipment cost and the need for trained sonographers limit its use in low-resource settings. The authors recruited 4,695 pregnant volunteers in North Carolina and Zambia and obtained blind ultrasound sweeps (cineloop videos) of the gravid abdomen alongside standard fetal biometry. They then trained a neural network to estimate gestational age from the sweeps and, in three test data sets, assessed the performance of the artificial intelligence model and biometry against previously established gestational age. The mean absolute error =/- standard error was 3.9±0.12 days for the model versus 4.7±0.15 days for biometry. The findings were supported in the test set of women who conceived by in vitro fertilization and in the set of women from whom sweeps were collected by untrained users with low-cost, battery-powered devices. Thus, the AI model estimated gestational age with accuracy similar to that of trained sonographers conducting standard fetal biometry. Performance of the model appeared to extend to blind sweeps collected by untrained providers in Zambia using low-cost devices.

Chapter 18. Orthopedics, rheumatology and sports medicine

- Convolutional neural networks for knee injuries[7]

Investigators developed three-dimensional convolutional neural networks to detect the regions of interest within magnetic resonance imaging studies of knee injuries and to grade abnormalities of the cartilage, bone marrow, menisci, and the anterior cruciate ligament. The area under the receiver operating characteristic curve for all tissues ranged from 0.83 to 0.93. The three-dimensional convolutional neural network had high sensitivity, specificity, and accuracy for knee-lesion-severity scoring and also increased intergrader agreement when used on an external dataset.

- An artificial intelligence decision support system, Aidoc, for the detection of cervical spinal fractures on non-contrast cervical spine CT scans and its poor performance

The study included 1,904 emergent non-contrast cervical spine CT scans of adult patients. The presence of cervical spinal fracture was determined by Aidoc and an attending neuroradiologist. Aidoc and the neuroradiologist's interpretation were concordant in 91.5% of cases. Aidoc correctly identified 67 of 122 fractures (54.9%) with 106 false-positive flagged studies. Diagnostic performance was calculated as the following: sensitivity, 54.9%; specificity, 94.1%; positive predictive value, 38.7%; and negative predictive value, 96.8%. Worsened performance was observed in the detection of chronic fractures. The authors concluded that there was poor diagnostic accuracy of this artificial intelligence decision support system for the detection of cervical spine fractures. Similar algorithms have also received little or no external validation, and this study raiseed concerns about their generalizability, utility, and rapid pace of deployment.

Chapter 19. Surgery

- Frozen section is widely used for intraoperative pathological diagnosis (IOPD), which is essential for intraoperative decision making. However, frozen section suffers from some drawbacks, such as being time consuming and having a high misdiagnosis rate.

The investigators hypothesized that AI with deep learning technology could help IOPD, with a computer trained by a large dataset of intraoperative lesion images.

The investigators concluded that real-time diagnosis, ease of use and high accuracy were potential advantages of AI for IOPD.[29]

Chapter 20. AI use in the Emergency Department

- AI is transforming the therapeutic relationship from the traditional physician-patient dyad into a triadic doctor-patient-machine relationship[61].

New AI technologies, however, require careful vetting, legal standards, patient safeguards, and provider education. Emergency physicians should recognize the limits and risks of AI as well as its potential benefits. They must learn to partner with, not capitulate to, AI. AI has proven to be superior to, or on a par with, certain physician skills, such as interpreting radiographs and making diagnoses based on visual cues, such as skin cancer. AI can provide cognitive assistance, but emergency physicians must interpret AI results within the clinical context of individual patients. They must also advocate for patient confidentiality, professional liability coverage, and the essential role of specialty-trained emergency physicians.

Chapter 21. AI use in the intensive care unit

The authors felt that the amount of data captured in the management of patients in an intensive care unit (ICU) was an ideal opportunity for exploiting the capabilities of AI.[65]

They described machine learning models that have been used in an ICU to predict pathologies (such as acute kidney injury), detect symptoms (including delirium), and propose therapeutic actions (such as the use of vasopressors and fluids in sepsis). They concluded that in the future, AI will be increasingly used in ICUs, due to the increasing quality and quantity of available data and the new AI technologies that will able to be harnessed to analyse these data.

Chapter 22. Drug-drug interactions (DDI)

The occurrence of DDI affects the treatment of patients and has become a serious problem for patient safety and drug management.[58,59] The harm caused by DDI will be greatly reduced if machine learning can be used to efficiently predict DDI. To this end, it is urgent to develop better-performing machine learning approaches. This article described existing machine learning-based approaches for predicting DDI. In the past 10 years, machine learning has been widely applied in bioinformatics and achieved good results. Under most of the existing approaches, drug similarity is taken as the most fundamental starting point for better prediction of DDI, assisted by a variety of other means. However, most current DDI predictions are limited to the interactions between two drugs. In the future work, the investigators will pursue the accuracy of predicting the probability of drug-drug interactions and the ability to accurately predict the types of drug-drug interactions. However, because the use of multiple drugs has become a trend in clinical medicine, it is urgent to develop methods to predict interactions between multiple drugs. In the opinion of the authors there are a number of ways to solve this problem which they predicted will be available in the near future.

Chapter 23. Concerns regarding the use of AI in healthcare

A major concern in making AI systems of practical value to large populations of patients is the ability of AI systems developed by one institution, or a group of institutions, to interact with, and be applicable to, the AI systems developed by other institutions or groups of institutions. This will likely need high-level governmental overview and mandatory instructions for AI systems to be compatible with each other. This may sound difficult to achieve, but comfort can be taken from the widespread use, and international acceptance of, systems such as MRI scans and other sophisticated diagnostic tools. In the case of MRI scans the issue was resolved by hospitals using the best, and cheapest, MRI scanners. A similar approach could be taken with AI healthcare systems.

Chapter 24. Conclusions and the future

This book examined peer-reviewed, published reports in the medical literature over the last five years on the use of AI applications to improve healthcare from 2016 to

2023 using AI systems before the availability of CHAT GPT4. We found abundant evidence of benefit. Many of these AI applications used machine learning on large numbers of images, illustrating the value that AI has added to interpretation of radiological images. It did not include articles using CHAT-GPT4, which is a large language-based AI software program announced in 2023 and which appears very promising.

A subsequent review of articles using CHAT GTP4 or similar software will be required to further assess the value of AI in healthcare. It is the authors' view that this area of medicine is in its early infancy.

References

1.Jones OT, Matin RN, van der Schaar M, Prathivadi Bhayankaram K, Ranmuthu CKI, Islam MS, Behiyat D, Boscott R, Calanzani N, Emery J, Williams HC, Walter FM. Artificial intelligence and machine learning algorithms for early detection of skin cancer in community and primary care settings: a systematic review. Lancet Digit Health. 2022 Jun;4(6):e466-e476. doi: 10.1016/S2589-7500(22)00023-1. PMID: 35623799.

2.Siontis KC, Noseworthy PA, Attia ZI, Friedman PA. Artificial intelligence-enhanced electrocardiography in cardiovascular disease management. Nat Rev Cardiol. 2021 Jul;18(7):465-478. doi: 10.1038/s41569-020-00503-2. Epub 2021 Feb 1. PMID: 33526938; PMCID: PMC7848866.

3.Lu MY, Chen TY, Williamson DFK, Zhao M, Shady M, Lipkova J, Mahmood F. AI-based pathology predicts origins for cancers of unknown primary. Nature. 2021 Jun;594(7861):106-110. doi: 10.1038/s41586-021-03512-4. Epub 2021 May 5. PMID: 33953404.

4.Yuan N, Kwan AC, Duffy G, Theurer J, Chen JH, Nieman K, Botting P, Dey D, Berman DS, Cheng S, Ouyang D. Prediction of Coronary Artery Calcium Using Deep Learning of Echocardiograms. J Am Soc Echocardiogr. 2023 May;36(5):474-481.e3. doi: 10.1016/j.echo.2022.12.014. Epub 2022 Dec 23. PMID: 36566995; PMCID: PMC10164107.

5.Sim Y, Chung MJ, Kotter E, Yune S, Kim M, Do S, Han K, Kim H, Yang S, Lee DJ, Choi BW. Deep Convolutional Neural Network-based Software Improves Radiologist Detection of Malignant Lung Nodules on Chest Radiographs. Radiology. 2020 Jan;294(1):199-209. doi: 10.1148/radiol.2019182465. Epub 2019 Nov 12. PMID: 31714194.

6.Eng D, Chute C, Khandwala N, Rajpurkar P, Long J, Shleifer S, Khalaf MH, Sandhu AT, Rodriguez F, Maron DJ, Seyyedi S, Marin D, Golub I, Budoff M, Kitamura F, Takahashi MS, Filice RW, Shah R, Mongan J, Kallianos K, Langlotz CP, Lungren MP, Ng AY, Patel BN. Automated coronary calcium scoring using deep learning with multicenter external validation. NPJ Digit Med. 2021 Jun 1;4(1):88. doi: 10.1038/s41746-021-00460-1. PMID: 34075194; PMCID: PMC8169744.

7.Astuto B, Flament I, K Namiri N, Shah R, Bharadwaj U, M Link T, D Bucknor M, Pedoia V, Majumdar S. Automatic Deep Learning-assisted Detection and Grading of Abnormalities in Knee MRI Studies. Radiol Artif Intell. 2021 Jan 20;3(3):e200165. doi: 10.1148/ryai.2021200165. Erratum in: Radiol Artif Intell. 2021 May 19;3(3):e219001. doi: 10.1148/ryai.2021219001. PMID: 34142088; PMCID: PMC8166108.

8.Tao Q, Yan W, Wang Y, Paiman EHM, Shamonin DP, Garg P, Plein S, Huang L, Xia L, Sramko M, Tintera J, de Roos A, Lamb HJ, van der Geest RJ. Deep Learning-based Method for Fully Automatic Quantification of Left Ventricle Function from Cine MR Images: A Multivendor, Multicenter Study. Radiology. 2019 Jan;290(1):81-88. doi: 10.1148/radiol.2018180513. Epub 2018 Oct 9. PMID: 30299231.

9.Elijovich L, Dornbos Iii D, Nickele C, Alexandrov A, Inoa-Acosta V, Arthur AS, Hoit D. Automated emergent large vessel occlusion detection by artificial intelligence improves stroke workflow in a hub and spoke stroke system of care. J Neurointerv Surg. 2022 Jul;14(7):704-708. doi: 10.1136/neurintsurg-2021-017714. Epub 2021 Aug 20. PMID: 34417344.

10.Hillis JM, Bizzo BC, Mercaldo S, Chin JK, Newbury-Chaet I, Digumarthy SR, Gilman MD, Muse VV, Bottrell G, Seah JCY, Jones CM, Kalra MK, Dreyer KJ. Evaluation of an Artificial Intelligence Model for Detection of Pneumothorax and Tension Pneumothorax in Chest Radiographs. JAMA Netw Open. 2022 Dec

1;5(12):e2247172. doi: 10.1001/jamanetworkopen.2022.47172. PMID: 36520432; PMCID: PMC9856508.

11.Pease M, Arefan D, Barber J, Yuh E, Puccio A, Hochberger K, Nwachuku E, Roy S, Casillo S, Temkin N, Okonkwo DO, Wu S; TRACK-TBI Investigators. Outcome Prediction in Patients with Severe Traumatic Brain Injury Using Deep Learning from Head CT Scans. Radiology. 2022 Aug;304(2):385-394. doi: 10.1148/radiol.212181. Epub 2022 Apr 26. PMID: 35471108; PMCID: PMC9340242.

12.Chin Lin, Wei-Ting Liu, Chiao-Hsiang Chang, Chiao-Chin Lee, Shi-Chue Hsing, Wen-Hui Fang, Dung-Jang. Artificial Intelligence–Powered Rapid Identification of ST-Elevation Myocardial Infarction via Electrocardiogram (ARISE) — A Pragmatic Randomized Controlled Trial. NEJM AI, June 24, 2024. doi10.1056/aioa2400190

13.European Society of Radiology (ESR). Current practical experience with artificial intelligence in clinical radiology: a survey of the European Society of Radiology. Insights Imaging 2022;13:107-107.

14.Allen B, Agarwal S, Coombs L, Wald C, Dreyer K. 2020 ACR Data Science Institute artificial intelligence survey. J Am Coll Radiol 2021;18:1153-1159.

15.Yuba M, Iwasaki K. Systematic analysis of the test design and performance of AI/ML-based medical devices approved for triage/detection/diagnosis in the USA and Japan. Sci Rep 2022;12:16874-16874.

16.Tariq A, Purkayastha S, Padmanaban GP, et al. Current clinical applications of artificial intelligence in radiology and their best supporting evidence. J Am Coll Radiol 2020;17:1371-1381.

17.Richardson ML, Garwood ER, Lee Y, et al. Noninterpretive uses of artificial intelligence in radiology. Acad Radiol 2021;28:1225-1235.

18.Wang G, Ye JC, De Man B. Deep learning for tomographic image reconstruction. Nat Mach Intell 2020;2:737-748.

19.Jiang Y, Zhang Z, Yuan Q, et al. Predicting peritoneal recurrence and disease-free survival from CT images in gastric cancer with multitask deep learning: a retrospective study. Lancet Digit Health 2022;4(5):e340-e350.

20.Karamchandani RR, Helms AM, Satyanarayana S, et al. Automated detection of intracranial large vessel occlusions using Viz.ai software: experience in a large, integrated stroke network. Brain Behav 2023;13(1):e2808-e2808.

21.Auffermann WF. AI Nodule Detection on Chest Radiographs Using Randomized Controlled Data: The Effect on Clinical Practice. Radiology. 2023 Apr;307(2):e223186. doi: 10.1148/radiol.223186. Epub 2023 Feb 7. PMID: 36749218.

22.Nam JG, Hwang EJ, Kim J, Park N, Lee EH, Kim HJ, Nam M, Lee JH, Park CM, Goo JM. AI Improves Nodule Detection on Chest Radiographs in a Health Screening Population: A Randomized Controlled Trial. Radiology. 2023 Apr;307(2):e221894. doi: 10.1148/radiol.221894. Epub 2023 Feb 7. PMID: 36749213.

23.Yoo H, Kim KH, Singh R, Digumarthy SR, Kalra MK. Validation of a Deep Learning Algorithm for the Detection of Malignant Pulmonary Nodules in Chest Radiographs. JAMA Netw Open. 2020 Sep 1;3(9):e2017135. doi: 10.1001/jamanetworkopen.2020.17135. PMID: 32970157; PMCID: PMC7516603.

24.Sim Y, Chung MJ, Kotter E, Yune S, Kim M, Do S, Han K, Kim H, Yang S, Lee DJ, Choi BW. Deep Convolutional Neural Network-based Software Improves Radiologist Detection of Malignant Lung Nodules on Chest Radiographs. Radiology. 2020 Jan;294(1):199-209. doi: 10.1148/radiol.2019182465. Epub 2019 Nov 12. PMID: 31714194.

25.Kitamura F, Takahashi MS, Filice RW, Shah R, Mongan J, Kallianos K, Langlotz CP, Lungren MP, Ng AY, Patel BN. Automated coronary calcium scoring using deep learning with multicenter external validation. NPJ Digit Med. 2021 Jun 1;4(1):88. doi: 10.1038/s41746-021-00460-1. PMID: 34075194; PMCID: PMC8169744.

26.Punjabi A, Martersteck A, Wang Y, Parrish TB, Katsaggelos AK; Alzheimer's Disease Neuroimaging Initiative. Neuroimaging modality fusion in Alzheimer's classification using convolutional neural networks. PLoS One. 2019 Dec 5;14(12):e0225759. doi: 10.1371/journal.pone.0225759. PMID: 31805160; PMCID: PMC6894831.

27.Kim HE, Kim HH, Han BK, Kim KH, Han K, Nam H, Lee EH, Kim EK. Changes in cancer detection and false-positive recall in mammography using artificial intelligence: a retrospective, multireader study. Lancet Digit Health. 2020 Mar;2(3):e138-e148. doi: 10.1016/S2589-7500(20)30003-0. Epub 2020 Feb 6. PMID: 33334578.

28.Brownstein, JS et al. Advances in Artificial Intelligence for Infectious-Disease Surveillance N Engl J Med 2023;388:1597-1607. DOI: 10.1056/NEJMra2119215

29.Zhang J, Song Y, Xia F, Zhu C, Zhang Y, Song W, Xu J, Ma X. Rapid and accurate intraoperative pathological diagnosis by artificial intelligence with deep learning technology. Med Hypotheses. 2017 Sep;107:98-99. doi: 10.1016/j.mehy.2017.08.021. Epub 2017 Sep 1. PMID: 28915974.

30.Wang P, Berzin TM, Glissen Brown JR, Bharadwaj S, Becq A, Xiao X, Liu P, Li L, Song Y, Zhang D, Li Y, Xu G, Tu M, Liu X. Real-time automatic detection system increases colonoscopic polyp and adenoma detection rates: a prospective randomised controlled study. Gut. 2019 Oct;68(10):1813-1819. doi: 10.1136/gutjnl-2018-317500. Epub 2019 Feb 27. PMID: 30814121; PMCID: PMC6839720.

31.Pak S, Park SG, Park J, Cho ST, Lee YG, Ahn H. Applications of artificial intelligence in urologic oncology. Investig Clin Urol. 2024 May;65(3):202-216. doi: 10.4111/icu.20230435. PMID: 38714511; PMCID: PMC11076794.

32.Suarez-Ibarrola R, Hein S, Reis G, Gratzke C, Miernik A. Current and future applications of machine and deep learning in urology: a review of the literature on urolithiasis, renal cell carcinoma, and bladder and prostate cancer. World J Urol. 2020 Oct;38(10):2329-2347. doi: 10.1007/s00345-019-03000-5. Epub 2019 Nov 5. PMID: 31691082.

33.Krause J, Gulshan V, Rahimy E, Karth P, Widner K, Corrado GS, Peng L, Webster DR. Grader Variability and the Importance of Reference Standards for Evaluating Machine Learning Models for Diabetic Retinopathy. Ophthalmology. 2018 Aug;125(8):1264-1272. doi: 10.1016/j.ophtha.2018.01.034. Epub 2018 Mar 13. PMID: 29548646.

34.Sayres R, Taly A, Rahimy E, Blumer K, Coz D, Hammel N, Krause J, Narayanaswamy A, Rastegar Z, Wu D, Xu S, Barb S, Joseph A, Shumski M, Smith J, Sood AB, Corrado GS, Peng L, Webster DR. Using a Deep Learning Algorithm and Integrated Gradients Explanation to Assist Grading for Diabetic Retinopathy.

Ophthalmology. 2019 Apr;126(4):552-564. doi: 10.1016/j.ophtha.2018.11.016. Epub 2018 Dec 13. PMID: 30553900.

35.Sayres R, Taly A, Rahimy E, Blumer K, Coz D, Hammel N, Krause J, Narayanaswamy A, Rastegar Z, Wu D, Xu S, Barb S, Joseph A, Shumski M, Smith J, Sood AB, Corrado GS, Peng L, Webster DR. Using a Deep Learning Algorithm and Integrated Gradients Explanation to Assist Grading for Diabetic Retinopathy. Ophthalmology. 2019 Apr;126(4):552-564. doi: 10.1016/j.ophtha.2018.11.016. Epub 2018 Dec 13. PMID: 30553900.

36.Gulshan V, Peng L, Coram M, Stumpe MC, Wu D, Narayanaswamy A, Venugopalan S, Widner K, Madams T, Cuadros J, Kim R, Raman R, Nelson PC, Mega JL, Webster DR. Development and Validation of a Deep Learning Algorithm for Detection of Diabetic Retinopathy in Retinal Fundus Photographs. JAMA. 2016 Dec 13;316(22):2402-2410. doi: 10.1001/jama.2016.17216. PMID: 27898976.

37.Chew EY, Burns SA, Abraham AG, Bakhoum MF, Beckman JA, Chui TYP, Finger RP, Frangi AF, Gottesman RF, Grant MB, Hanssen H, Lee CS, Meyer ML, Rizzoni D, Rudnicka AR, Schuman JS, Seidelmann SB, Tang WHW, Adhikari BB, Danthi N, Hong Y, Reid D, Shen GL, Oh YS. Standardization and clinical applications of retinal imaging biomarkers for cardiovascular disease: a Roadmap from an NHLBI workshop. Nat Rev Cardiol. 2024 Jul 22. doi: 10.1038/s41569-024-01060-8. Epub ahead of print. PMID: 39039178.

38.Steiner DF, MacDonald R, Liu Y, Truszkowski P, Hipp JD, Gammage C, Thng F, Peng L, Stumpe MC. Impact of Deep Learning Assistance on the Histopathologic Review of Lymph Nodes for Metastatic Breast Cancer. Am J Surg Pathol. 2018 Dec;42(12):1636-1646. doi: 10.1097/PAS.0000000000001151. PMID: 30312179; PMCID: PMC6257102.

39.Ehteshami Bejnordi B, et al. Diagnostic Assessment of Deep Learning Algorithms for Detection of Lymph Node Metastases in Women With Breast Cancer. JAMA. 2017 Dec 12;318(22):2199-2210. doi: 10.1001/jama.2017.14585. PMID: 29234806; PMCID: PMC5820737.

40.Chilamkurthy S, Ghosh R, Tanamala S, Biviji M, Campeau NG, Venugopal VK, Mahajan V, Rao P, Warier P. Deep learning algorithms for detection of critical findings in head CT scans: a retrospective study. Lancet. 2018 Dec 1;392(10162):2388-2396. doi: 10.1016/S0140-6736(18)31645-3. Epub 2018 Oct 11. PMID: 30318264.

41.Yeo M, Tahayori B, Kok HK, Maingard J, Kutaiba N, Russell J, Thijs V, Jhamb A, Chandra RV, Brooks M, Barras CD, Asadi H. Evaluation of techniques to improve a deep learning algorithm for the automatic detection of intracranial hemorrhage on CT head imaging. Eur Radiol Exp. 2023 Apr 10;7(1):17. doi: 10.1186/s41747-023-00330-3. PMID: 37032417; PMCID: PMC10083149.

42.Galloway, CD et al. Non-invasive detection of hyperkalemia with a smartphone electrocardiogram and artificial intelligence. Journal of the American College of Cardiology, 2018, Vol.71(11), p.A272-A272. DOI: 10.1016/S0735-1097(18)30813-1.

43.Esteva A, Kuprel B, Novoa RA, Ko J, Swetter SM, Blau HM, Thrun S. Dermatologist-level classification of skin cancer with deep neural networks. Nature. 2017 Feb 2;542(7639):115-118. doi: 10.1038/nature21056. Epub 2017 Jan 25. Erratum in: Nature. 2017 Jun 28;546(7660):686. doi: 10.1038/nature22985. PMID: 28117445; PMCID: PMC8382232.

44.Wilson M, Chopra R, Wilson MZ, Cooper C, MacWilliams P, Liu Y, Wulczyn E, Florea D, Hughes CO, Karthikesalingam A, Khalid H, Vermeirsch S, Nicholson L, Keane PA, Balaskas K, Kelly CJ. Validation and Clinical Applicability of Whole-Volume Automated Segmentation of Optical Coherence Tomography in Retinal Disease Using Deep Learning. JAMA Ophthalmol. 2021 Sep 1;139(9):964-973. doi: 10.1001/jamaophthalmol.2021.2273. PMID: 34236406; PMCID: PMC8444027.

45.Lee HW, Jin KN, Oh S, Kang SY, Lee SM, Jeong IB, Son JW, Han JH, Heo EY, Lee JG, Kim YJ, Kim EY, Cho YJ. Artificial Intelligence Solution for Chest Radiographs in Respiratory Outpatient Clinics: Multicenter Prospective Randomized Clinical Trial. Ann Am Thorac Soc. 2023 May;20(5):660-667. doi: 10.1513/AnnalsATS.202206-481OC. PMID: 36508316.

46.Rueckel J, Kunz WG, Hoppe BF, Patzig M, Notohamiprodjo M, Meinel FG, Cyran CC, Ingrisch M, Ricke J, Sabel BO. Artificial Intelligence Algorithm Detecting Lung Infection in Supine Chest Radiographs of Critically ill Patients With a Diagnostic

Accuracy Similar to Board-Certified Radiologists. Crit Care Med. 2020 Jul;48(7):e574-e583. doi: 10.1097/CCM.0000000000004397. PMID: 32433121.

47.Bai HX, Wang R, Xiong Z, Hsieh B, Chang K, Halsey K, Tran TML, Choi JW, Wang DC, Shi LB, Mei J, Jiang XL, Pan I, Zeng QH, Hu PF, Li YH, Fu FX, Huang RY, Sebro R, Yu QZ, Atalay MK, Liao WH. Artificial Intelligence Augmentation of Radiologist Performance in Distinguishing COVID-19 from Pneumonia of Other Origin at Chest CT. Radiology. 2020 Sep;296(3):E156-E165. doi: 10.1148/radiol.2020201491. Epub 2020 Apr 27. Erratum in: Radiology. 2021 Apr;299(1):E225. doi: 10.1148/radiol.2021219004. PMID: 32339081; PMCID: PMC7233483.

48.Pokaprakarn T, Prieto JC, Price JT, Kasaro MP, Sindano N, Shah HR, Peterson M, Akapelwa MM, Kapilya FM, Sebastião YV, Goodnight W 3rd, Stringer EM, Freeman BL, Montoya LM, Chi BH, Rouse DJ, Cole SR, Vwalika B, Kosorok MR, Stringer JSA. AI Estimation of Gestational Age from Blind Ultrasound Sweeps in Low-Resource Settings. NEJM Evid. 2022 May;1(5):10.1056/evidoa2100058. doi: 10.1056/evidoa2100058. Epub 2022 Mar 28. PMID: 36875289; PMCID: PMC9980216.

49.Hsu W, Hippe DS, Nakhaei N, Wang PC, Zhu B, Siu N, Ahsen ME, Lotter W, Sorensen AG, Naeim A, Buist DSM, Schaffter T, Guinney J, Elmore JG, Lee CI. External Validation of an Ensemble Model for Automated Mammography Interpretation by Artificial Intelligence. JAMA Netw Open. 2022 Nov 1;5(11):e2242343. doi: 10.1001/jamanetworkopen.2022.42343. PMID: 36409497; PMCID: PMC9679879.

50.Al Badawy EA, Saha A, Mazurowski MA. Deep learning for segmentation of brain tumors: Impact of cross-institutional training and testing. Med Phys. 2018 Mar;45(3):1150-1158. doi: 10.1002/mp.12752. Epub 2018 Feb 8. PMID: 29356028.

51.Voter AF, Larson ME, Garrett JW, Yu JJ. Diagnostic Accuracy and Failure Mode Analysis of a Deep Learning Algorithm for the Detection of Cervical Spine Fractures. AJNR Am J Neuroradiol. 2021 Aug;42(8):1550-1556. doi: 10.3174/ajnr.A7179. Epub 2021 Jun 11. PMID: 34117018; PMCID: PMC8367597.

52.Park A, Chute C, Rajpurkar P, Lou J, Ball RL, Shpanskaya K, Jabarkheel R, Kim LH, McKenna E, Tseng J, Ni J, Wishah F, Wittber F, Hong DS, Wilson TJ, Halabi S, Basu S, Patel BN, Lungren MP, Ng AY, Yeom KW. Deep Learning-Assisted Diagnosis of Cerebral Aneurysms Using the HeadXNet Model. JAMA Netw Open. 2019 Jun 5;2(6):e195600. doi: 10.1001/jamanetworkopen.2019.5600. PMID: 31173130; PMCID: PMC6563570.

53.Rajpurkar P, O'Connell C, Schechter A, Asnani N, Li J, Kiani A, Ball RL, Mendelson M, Maartens G, van Hoving DJ, Griesel R, Ng AY, Boyles TH, Lungren MP. CheXaid: deep learning assistance for physician diagnosis of tuberculosis using chest x-rays in patients with HIV. NPJ Digit Med. 2020 Sep 9;3:115. doi: 10.1038/s41746-020-00322-2. PMID: 32964138; PMCID: PMC7481246.

54.Panch T, Mattie H, Celi LA. The "inconvenient truth" about AI in healthcare. NPJ Digit Med. 2019 Aug 16;2:77. doi: 10.1038/s41746-019-0155-4. PMID: 31453372; PMCID: PMC6697674.

55.Feng J, Phillips RV, Malenica I, Bishara A, Hubbard AE, Celi LA, Pirracchio R. Clinical artificial intelligence quality improvement: towards continual monitoring and updating of AI algorithms in healthcare. NPJ Digit Med. 2022 May 31;5(1):66. doi: 10.1038/s41746-022-00611-y. PMID: 35641814; PMCID: PMC9156743.

56.Huang SC, Pareek A, Zamanian R, Banerjee I, Lungren MP. Multimodal fusion with deep neural networks for leveraging CT imaging and electronic health record: a case-study in pulmonary embolism detection. Sci Rep. 2020 Dec 17;10(1):22147. doi: 10.1038/s41598-020-78888-w. PMID: 33335111; PMCID: PMC7746687.

58.Remy-Jardin M, Faivre JB, Kaergel R, Hutt A, Felloni P, Khung S, Lejeune AL, Giordano J, Remy J. Machine Learning and Deep Neural Network Applications in the Thorax: Pulmonary Embolism, Chronic Thromboembolic Pulmonary Hypertension, Aorta, and Chronic Obstructive Pulmonary Disease. J Thorac Imaging. 2020 May;35 Suppl 1:S40-S48. doi: 10.1097/RTI.0000000000000492. PMID: 32271281

59.Han K, Cao P, Wang Y, Xie F, Ma J, Yu M, Wang J, Xu Y, Zhang Y, Wan J. A Review of Approaches for Predicting Drug-Drug Interactions Based on Machine Learning. Front Pharmacol. 2022 Jan 28;12:814858. doi: 10.3389/fphar.2021.814858. PMID: 35153767; PMCID: PMC8835726.

60.Zhang Y, Deng Z, Xu X, Feng Y, Junliang S. Application of Artificial Intelligence in Drug-Drug Interactions Prediction: A Review. J Chem Inf Model. 2024 Apr 8;64(7):2158-2173. doi: 10.1021/acs.jcim.3c00582. Epub 2023 Jul 17. PMID: 37458400.

61.Lee P, Bubeck S, Petro J. Benefits, Limits, and Risks of GPT-4 as an AI Chatbot for Medicine. N Engl J Med. 2023 Mar 30;388(13):1233-1239. doi: 10.1056/NEJMsr2214184. PMID: 36988602.

62.Vearrier L, Derse AR, Basford JB, Larkin GL, Moskop JC. Artificial Intelligence in Emergency Medicine: Benefits, Risks, and Recommendations. J Emerg Med. 2022 Apr;62(4):492-499. doi: 10.1016/j.jemermed.2022.01.001. Epub 2022 Feb 11. PMID: 35164977.

63.Kermany DS, Goldbaum M, Cai W, Valentim CCS, Liang H, Baxter SL, McKeown A, Yang G, Wu X, Yan F, Dong J, Prasadha MK, Pei J, Ting MYL, Zhu J, Li C, Hewett S, Dong J, Ziyar I, Shi A, Zhang R, Zheng L, Hou R, Shi W, Fu X, Duan Y, Huu VAN, Wen C, Zhang ED, Zhang CL, Li O, Wang X, Singer MA, Sun X, Xu J, Tafreshi A, Lewis MA, Xia H, Zhang K. Identifying Medical Diagnoses and Treatable Diseases by Image-Based Deep Learning. Cell. 2018 Feb 22;172(5):1122-1131.e9. doi: 10.1016/j.cell.2018.02.010. PMID: 29474911.

64.Poplin R, Varadarajan AV, Blumer K, Liu Y, McConnell MV, Corrado GS, Peng L, Webster DR. Prediction of cardiovascular risk factors from retinal fundus photographs via deep learning. Nat Biomed Eng. 2018 Mar;2(3):158-164. doi: 10.1038/s41551-018-0195-0. Epub 2018 Feb 19. PMID: 31015713.

65.Mori Y, Kudo SE, Misawa M, Saito Y, Ikematsu H, Hotta K, Ohtsuka K, Urushibara F, Kataoka S, Ogawa Y, Maeda Y, Takeda K, Nakamura H, Ichimasa K, Kudo T, Hayashi T, Wakamura K, Ishida F, Inoue H, Itoh H, Oda M, Mori K. Real-Time Use of Artificial Intelligence in Identification of Diminutive Polyps During Colonoscopy: A Prospective Study. Ann Intern Med. 2018 Sep 18;169(6):357-366. doi: 10.7326/M18-0249. Epub 2018 Aug 14. PMID: 30105375.

66.Greco M, Caruso PF, Cecconi M. Artificial Intelligence in the Intensive Care Unit. Semin Respir Crit Care Med. 2021 Feb;42(1):2-9. doi: 10.1055/s-0040-1719037. Epub 2020 Nov 5. PMID: 33152770.

Made in the USA
Monee, IL
05 November 2026

67380846R00071